NATURAL REMEDIES

NATURAL
REMEDIES

*Techniques for
Preventing Headaches
and the Common Cold*

Norman D. Ford

Galahad Books . New York

Previously published in two volumes as EIGHTEEN NATURAL WAYS TO BEAT A HEADACHE, Copyright © 1990 by Norman D. Ford and EIGHTEEN NATURAL WAYS TO BEAT THE COMMON COLD, Copyright © 1987 by Norman D. Ford.

First Galahad Books edition published in 1995.

Galahad Books
A division of Budget Book Service, Inc.
386 Park Avenue South
New York, NY 10016

Galahad Books is a registered trademark of Budget Book Service, Inc.

Published by arrangement with Keats Publishing, Inc.

Library of Congress Catalog Card Number 94-74487

ISBN: 0-88365-901-8

Printed in the United States of America.

11.45

Contents

NATURAL
HEADACHE REMEDIES

Contents

Acknowledgments

Most of the research behind this book was derived from some of America's most distinguished university medical centers and from such leading health advisory agencies as the National Institutes of Health, the American Heart Association, the National Academy of Sciences, and the Public Citizen Health Research Group. Virtually all of these studies support the validity and effectiveness of a multi-disciplinary approach to healing, and of the various alternative healing therapies described in this book.

So many sources were consulted in researching this book that it is impractical to acknowledge every one. However, I would like to acknowledge my debt to the research carried out by James Breneman M.D., Chairman, Allergy Committee, American Academy of Allergists; David E Bresler, Ph.D., director, Bresler Pain Center, Los Angeles; David R. Coddon, director, Headache Clinic, Mount Sinai Medical Center, New York; Seymour Diamond, M.D., director, Diamond Headache Clinic and National Migraine Foundation, Chicago; Arthur Elkind, M.D., director, Elkind Headache Clinic, Mount Vernon, New York; Arnold P. Friedman, M.D., founder, Montefiore Headache Unit, New York; Elmer E. Green, Ph.D., Menninger Foundation Biofeedback and Psycho-Physiology Center, Topeka, Kansas; Scott Haldeman, Ph.D., assistant clinical professor of neurology, University of California, Irvine; Robert S. Kunkel, M.D., director, Cleveland Clinic Headache Center; James Lance, M.D., University of New South Wales, Australia; Joan Millep, Ph.D., director, Atlanta Headache Clinic; Michael Moskowitz, M.D., Harvard University Medical School; Neil Raskin, M.D., professor of neurology, University of California, San Fran-

cisco; Joel R. Saper, M.D., director, Michigan Headache
and Neurological Institute; C. Norman Sheeley M.D., Pain
and Health Rehabilitation Center, La Crosse, Wisconsin;
Patricia Solbach, Ph.D., research psychologist, Menninger
Clinic, Topeka, Kansas; John E. Upledger, Ph.D., former
director, Unity Holistic Health Center, West Palm Beach,
Florida; American Association for the Study of Headache,
San Clemente, California; National Headache Foundation,
Chicago; National Migraine Foundation, Chicago; Califor-
nia Medical Clinic for Headache, Encino, California; Faulker
Headache Research Center, Boston; Houston Headache
Clinic, Houston; City of London Migraine Clinic, London,
England; UCLA Pain Management Center, Los Angeles.

Several short passages in Chapter 9 are quoted from the
author's companion book in this series, *Eighteen Natural
Ways to Beat the Common Cold*, Keats Publishing, Inc.,
1987.

1 The Drugless Way to Headache Relief

The snapping open of medicine cabinet doors as we reach inside for a pill to relieve a headache has become one of the most familiar sounds on the American scene.

Which is hardly surprising when you consider that TV ads bombard us with messages to reach for a pill for every ill. Altogether, we hand over more than two billion dollars annually for over the counter (OTC) and prescription drugs for headache relief.

Today, a huge multi-billion-dollar pharmaceutical and advertising industry has evolved, dedicated to conditioning us to believe that headaches can be cured only by a chemically active drug. For people who get only an occasional, simple tension headache, this is probably true. But what happens when two aspirin aren't enough?

All too many chronic headaches defy aspirin, and stronger painkillers are needed to dull the pain. Every drug is a two-edged sword; the pharmaceutical benefits are very often offset by adverse side effects. And the side effects of many headache drugs are so destructive that, at most headache clinics, the first step is to get new patients off all painkilling drugs, and then off any other non-essential medications, as swiftly as possible.

DRUGS MAY CAUSE MORE HEADACHES THAN THEY CURE

One reason is that so many chronic headache sufferers tend to take two or more medications on a daily basis. In 1984, at the New England Center for Headache in Greenwich, Connecticut (it has since moved to Stamford), a study was made on patients who took several different painkillers each day for their chronic headache pain. The drugs were gradually withdrawn altogether. After being drug-free for one month, 66 percent of the patients reported significantly fewer headaches and, after a second month, the number had grown to 81 percent.

At least half their headaches had been caused by the very drugs they were taking to try and relieve their headache pain.

Another reason why clinics immediately phase out painkilling drugs is that, even at recommended dosages, addiction to both OTC and prescription drugs can easily occur.

BREAKING THE BONDAGE OF DRUGS

According to a report in the National Headache Foundation's newsletter, fall, 1988, Arthur H. Elkind, M.D., director of the Elkind Headache Clinic in Mount Vernon, New York, stated at a national headache conference that many people with chronic headaches use excessive amounts of prescription and OTC medications for relief.

Drug dependency is common. Among medications that Dr. Elkind found most frequently abused were not only potent prescription drugs like ergotamine, barbiturates and codeine, but OTC analgesics containing aspirin or acet-aminophen, often in combination with caffeine.

We're not trying to exaggerate the risks of common OTC headache medications. People generally know that two aspirin will relieve most acute tension headaches within half an hour without causing adverse side effects. Yet a rule of thumb in most headache clinics is that if two aspirin don't relieve a headache within thirty minutes, taking more aspirin isn't likely to help.

A PILL FOR EVERY ILL

Most of us are so accustomed to assuming that a drug or injection exists to provide instant relief for almost any kind of pain, that we tend to see a drug solution for just about every problem.

This has led most Americans to severely overestimate the curative power of headache drugs. The cold facts are that, for other than the occasional mild tension headache, most anti-headache drugs are only 70 percent effective in providing relief. And no really dependable drug exists for treating cluster or menstrual migraine headaches.

Furthermore, studies have shown that approximately 33 percent of the benefits ascribed to headache medications are due, not to any pharmaceutical action, but to the placebo effect—to the patient's own belief in the drug's ability to heal. When we subtract the healing power of the placebo effect, it is only too apparent that drug therapy has severe limitations of which most people are unaware.

A PHARMACOPOEIA OF HARSH AND DANGEROUS DRUGS

Every drug, to some extent, is toxic to the human body, so much so that doctors speak in terms of how well a certain drug is tolerated. Even at recommended doses, most drugs are mildly poisonous. For example, aspirin is so toxic that it can cause irritation or bleeding in the stomach and intestines, while continued use may erode the intestinal lining and form an ulcer. Common side effects of other headache drugs range from nausea to drowsiness, dizziness, confusion, bone loss, depression, vivid night-mares, insomnia, forgetfulness, breathing difficulties, rash and itching, hallucinations, blurred vision, dry mouth, kidney problems and even stroke.

However, virtually every headache specialist agrees that drugs may be essential for treating unusually stubborn cases of chronic headache. In severe cases of migraine and cluster headaches, a combination of drug and non-drug therapies may have to be used until the drugs can eventually be phased out.

But beyond these exceptions, the benefits of drug treat-ment often do *not* outweigh the risk of harm from adverse side effects. To some degree, most drugs are both carcino-genic and immunosuppressive, meaning that they may increase long-term risk of cancer and infections. Other headache drugs may increase risk of heart attack. It is widespread national concern about the disturbing side ef-fects of these drugs that has renewed interest in non-drug ways to overcome headache.

All over America, the hazards and low efficacy of drug-focused headache treatment are promoting a renaissance for alternative health care therapies, a movement which is gaining increasing support from the health care profession-als who staff the nation's headache and pain clinics.

HEADACHE CLINICS BEAT CHRONIC HEADACHES WITH DRUGLESS MEDICINE

Almost unknown to both doctors and the general public is the existance of some 25 medical clinics that specialize in headaches. In addition, several hundred medically operated pain clinics also treat headache pain. Many are associated with university medical centers and are manned by licensed health professionals from a variety of disciplines. These headache specialists have demonstrated a remarkable track record in achieving permanent relief from all types of headaches without drugs or other forms of mainstream medical treatment.

Although the clinics do employ drugs in extremely stubborn cases, the consensus of most headache specialists is that drugs are inappropriate for headache relief and that only natural, nonmedical therapies can permanently relieve most chronic headache pain.

Working with this philosophy, researchers at major headache clinics have made astonishing strides in developing natural, drugless therapies that relieve painful headaches, even when all other forms of treatment have failed. The anti-headache techniques used by these clinics employ do-it-yourself methods that almost anyone can use at home, usually without special know-how or equipment. The purpose of this book is to describe each of these anti-headache techniques so that you can begin to use them to treat your own headache pain.

STRESS IS THE UNDERLYING CAUSE OF MOST HEADACHES

Contributing to the success of most headache clinics is the growing recognition that stress is the underlying cause of the majority of headaches. This is hardly surprising since medical science now recognizes that virtually every disorder is stress-related, at least to some extent. Unresolved emotional stress is generally considered to be the underlying cause of at least 80 per cent of headaches, with the remainder being due to a variety of other forms of stress, ranging from the physical stress of noise or flickering lights, to the biological stress of low blood sugar.

Lack of funding, and difficulty in correlating stress to headaches in a laboratory setting, account for the paucity of documented evidence supporting the stress origin of headaches in medical journals. Compared to the $250 million awarded to research diabetes in 1989, the National Institute of Neurological Disorders and Stroke allotted a mere $1.4 million for headache research. Nonetheless, among headache specialists themselves, there is wide clinical acceptance of stress as the underlying cause of most headaches.

For example, *U.S. News* (July 31, 1989, page 4) begins its major coverage report on headaches by saying, "Stress has long been considered the principal cause of all headaches." And Arnold Fox, M.D. and Barry Fox, Ph.D., authors of *The Beverly Hills Diet*, recently advised in *Let's Live* Magazine (September 1989, page 59) that we should "start attacking the number one cause of headaches: stress."

Migraines are no exception. Discussing migraine trigger mechanisms, the Migraine Foundation of Toronto, Canada, states in its literature, "Migraine is triggered by precipitating or provoking factors—elements of stress, whether physical, emotional or situational that, given the predisposition, set off the actual headache process." The same literature notes that stress can consist of worry, anxiety, tension, emotional change, excitement, shock, repressed hostility, anger or depression, all arising from life situations.

Again, Dr. Seymour Diamond, director of the Diamond Headache Clinic and National Migraine Foundation, Chicago, stated recently that, "Our modern world is rampant with tension, frustration, anxiety, depression and repressed hostility, all of which can trigger headache pain. A multitude of chronic, recurring headaches are precipitated by stress."

And in his headache classic, *Headaches, The Drugless*

Way to Lasting Relief (Celestial Arts, 1987), Harry C. Ehrmantraut, Ph.D. states, "As a general rule, it is safe to say that a tension headache is precipitated by tension in the immediate life situation. This may arise from anger, aggravation, frustration, guilt or related emotional states."

Several authorities believe that marital stress is one of the most common causes of headaches. To confirm this, Rajan Roy, Ph.D., associate professor of social work and psychiatry at the University of Manitoba, studied 15 married couples. In each marriage, one partner suffered from recurrent tension or migraine headaches and all were experiencing marital stress. After a series of counseling sessions designed to reduce marital stress, 11 of the headache sufferers reported that their headaches were vastly improved.

Certainly, headaches can be provoked by drugs, illness, alcohol or other causes. But the prevailing opinion of most headache specialists is that the majority of headaches are provoked by negative emotions arising out of conflicts concerning job, money, marriage or similar life situations.

HEADACHES ARE A WHOLE PERSON DYSFUNCTION

Another reason that headache clinics have been eminently successful is that their treatment methods are based on the Whole Person or holistic approach. This is logical since almost all headaches begin with emotional stress that is translated into physiological mechanisms. Pain occurs as arteries in the head dilate. But the pain itself can only be experienced in the brain.

A headache is, therefore, a Whole Person phenomenon that involves the physical, mental, emotional, attitudinal, cognitive and even the nutritional and spiritual levels of the body-mind. Headache clinics respond to this Whole Person involvement by employing an array of alternative healing therapies which work on varying levels of body-mind function.

Doctors have attempted to duplicate the holistic approach by using a "background" drug as a daily prophylactic, and then using painkilling drugs whenever a headache occurs. As might be expected, this shotgun approach serves only to multiply side effects to the point where patients become increasingly depressed, helpless and dependent on drugs.

What most of us fail to recognize is that drugs often only duplicate tasks that the body-mind itself is entirely capable of doing in a normally healthy person.

In most cases, by using the natural therapies in this book, we may restore lost functions to the point where drugs are no longer needed. Our bodymind then becomes capable of taking over the job once more.

The Whole Person approach to healing is also known as holistic healing or holistic medicine. In medical science, its equivalent is behavioral medicine, a multi-disciplinary approach which employs multi-modal therapies. This means that behavioral medicine is administered by M.D.s. Although able to prescribe strong drugs should they be needed, behaviorial physicians prefer to minimize the use of pharmaceuticals, and most employ drugs only when absolutely essential. Much preferred are harmless, non-drug therapies such as acupuncture, acupressure, nutrition, massage exercise, heat and cold therapy, relaxation, biofeedback, creative imagery, stress management and cognitive positivism.

SELF-HELP FOR YOUR HEADACHE

Each of these natural therapies is widely used by headache and pain clinics and, of course, each is also freely available for anyone to use. By using a holistic approach, that is, using therapies that function on several different mindbody levels simultaneously, we can practice Behavioral Medicine on our own. By using several different natural therapies—for example, one physical, one nutritional and one cognitive—we can often intervene in our own headache with far greater success than by using drugs.

Natural therapies are classified as either active or passive. Active therapies are the core of behavioral medicine. By forcing us to take an active role in our own recovery, active therapies promote taking control of our lives and taking responsibility for our own wellness.

Among active therapies are attitudinal and cognitive therapies, exercise, relaxation, biofeedback, creative imagery, nutrition, heat and cold therapy, self-massage, acupressure, stretching and breathing techniques, identifying nutritional and environmental headache triggers, and do-it-yourself homeopathy and herbal medicine. Each encourages us to take action in response to our pain and stress and so to help ourselves.

This book can't exercise for you, relax for you, make images in your mind, or reprogram the beliefs that are causing your headaches. Behavioral medicine puts you in control and it's up to you to take an active role.

Among passive therapies are acupuncture, massage, homeopathy and herbal medicine prescribed by others as well as all drug medications. In each, something is *done to us* by a substance or by a person. While passive therapies can provide useful short-term relief, a holistic array of more active therapies is usually required to reverse the underlying cause of chronic headache pain.

HOLISTIC HEALING: THE NEW AGE MEDICINE

With all these options available, the drugless treatments you choose will be those that seem most appropriate for you and for your particular type of headache. Whichever you choose, we strongly recommend that you thoroughly read chapters 1, 2, and 3, which have to do with the attitudinal approach to anti-headache techniques.

For instance, the present chapter, Chapter 1, motivates you to minimize dependence on nonessential headache drugs. Chapter 2 urges you to obtain medical assurance that your headache is benign. And Chapter 3 describes how to gain power over your headache by becoming a medically informed layperson. Together, these chapters form the backbone of any Whole Person approach to permanent relief from chronic headache.

To play an active role in your own recovery from headaches—or any other dysfunction—you must know how to act and what to do. Thus the first step in practicing holistic healing is to acquire this know-how. By the time you have read and absorbed Chapters 1, 2, and 3, you will probably know more about headaches than your doctor does. Chapter by chapter, you should then read and absorb the remainder of this book. It is not a large book and a good reader can easily finish it in a single evening.

You will find that each chapter expands your knowledge of headaches and adds to the number of alternative therapies you can use.

We also very strongly urge that, as part of your holistic healing program, you include Anti-Headache Technique #17, **Liberate Yourself from Headaches With Cognitive Positivism.** For this is the *only* modality that can actually help rid us of the underlying cause of headaches.

Among other options, we recommend choosing one or more techniques from as many chapters as you can. Each chapter describes a group of therapies all of which function on a common approach. For instance, to relieve and banish chronic tension headache, you might choose these anti-headache techniques:

7-A, A Simple Stretching Technique.
12, Temperature Therapy for Speedy Relief.
14, Deep Relaxation With Muscle Tensing.
When these techniques, incorporating the physical and relaxation approaches, are coupled with Chapters 1, 2 and 3 and Technique #17, they offer a truly holistic approach.

To relieve and eventually banish chronic migraine, you might choose to employ these anti-headache techniques:

5, Headache Freedom Through Tryptophan Loading
6, Herbal Relief for Migraine Pain.
14 & 15, Deep Relaxation and Biofeedback.
These techniques use the nutritional, herbal and relaxation approaches. Together with Chapters 1, 2 and 3 and Technique #17, they also offer a truly holistic approach.

MINIMIZE DEPENDENCY ON NONESSENTIAL DRUGS

The focus of this chapter is on *minimizing dependency* on nonessential headache medications. It is not intended to dissuade you from taking drugs prescribed by your doctor, or drugs which may be essential to your health.

With this caveat in mind, the first step in freeing yourself from headaches is to take a cue from the headache clinics. Their prime concern is to get patients off painkillers as quickly as possible, and then off any other drugs.

If you are taking a prescription drug, or an OTC drug on your doctor's recommendation, or are under medical treatment for any reason at all, you must seek your doctor's approval and cooperation before reducing the dosage, and phasing out, any drug. Drugs prescribed for dysfunctions such as hypertension or heart disease may also precipitate chronic headaches. Your doctor may consider such drugs to be essential.

Even if your doctor does agree to phase out a drug, you

may have to do it under medical supervision because you may already be addicted to the drug.

GETTING FREE OF THE MEDICAL STRAITJACKET

If your physician is the type who overmedicalizes everything and attempts to solve all problems with drugs, you may want to seek a second medical opinion. Some physicians will prescribe a drug even when the problem is one for which drugs are not the best answer. When a side effect appears, they tend to view it as a brand new disease to be treated by prescribing yet another drug.

It would be wise to seek a second opinion about any decision to "manage" your headache with drugs on a long-term basis. This is especially important if you are taking a daily "background" drug and add a painkiller during attacks. It is all too possible that, far from being the best treatment for your condition, such drug management has been prescribed as the treatment least likely to provoke a litigation suit.

Side effects from "maintenance" drugs have turned many chronic headache sufferers into passive, helpless zombies. If you suspect you are being kept on a drug that you may not really need, you should seek a second medical opinion. Not all doctors are equally competent. Even within medicine, there is a choice of regimes for treating chronic headache. A second doctor may know of a less costly, less harmful, and more effective treatment of which your own doctor is unaware.

BACKLASH AGAINST PHARMACEUTICALS

One reason headache medications may fail to work is that the majority were originally developed for treating other diseases. While medical science has focused its efforts on finding a cure for killer diseases like cancer and heart disease, research into the causes and cure of headaches has been ignored. Primarily, this is because headaches are not usually life-threatening.

In 1987, the National Institutes of Health spent only $932,000 on headache research compared to over $500 million on heart disease. The result is that few drugs have been developed primarily for headache relief; and as far as curing chronic headaches goes, the other drugs don't appear to be getting the job done.

Headache drugs are classified as either abortive painkilling drugs or as prophylactic drugs.

Abortive Painkilling Drugs

Chief among these are the nonsteroidal anti-inflammatory drugs (NSAIDs) which inhibit synthesis of prostaglandins, hormone-like substances essential to the headache process. The principal NSAIDs include aspirin, acetaminophen and ibuprofen, all available OTC. These drugs work best on tension headaches.

Besides causing irritation or bleeding in stomach and intestines, continued use of aspirin may erode the intestinal lining and cause an ulcer. It can also impair blood coagulation, increase the tendency to bleed, lead to a higher risk of iron-deficiency anemia in younger women, and increase risk of a bleeding-type stroke. Nor are acetaminophen or ibuprofen panaceas. Each has a discouraging list of adverse side effects.

Once migraine begins, it can be stopped only by a powerful vasoconstrictor like ergotamine, a drug so fraught with side effects that it is prescribed only for severe migraine or cluster headache. Even then, it can be used only periodically. The steroid prednisone, occasionally prescribed to halt a cluster headache bout, has such a list of severe adverse side effects that it is used only when all else has failed.

Painkilling cocktails that often include codeine, tranquilizers or barbiturates are also commonly prescribed. All are addictive, and they are much overused. The analgesic lidocaine, another heart disease drug prescribed to relieve cluster headache, also carries a long list of adverse side effects.

Prophylactic Drugs

Prophylactic drugs are prescribed on a long-term basis to prevent headaches from occurring. Most carry risk of severe side effects and habitual dependency. Both beta blockers and calcium channel blockers are heart disease drugs, prescribed to reduce the severity and frequency of migraine and cluster headaches. Beta blockers work by blocking receptors in blood vessels to prevent constriction by norepinephrine. Calcium channel blockers achieve the same effect by blocking calcium uptake into muscles surrounding blood vessel walls. Both are addictive, may lead to constipation and drowsiness, and have a melancholy list of other adverse side effects.

Antidepressants are also prescribed when tension headaches seem due to depression or anxiety. They prevent uptake of serotonin into nerve cells, thus freeing existing serotonin to function as a neurotransmitter. Curiously, one of the many adverse side effects of these drugs is to heighten motivation for suicide, the very thing the drug is supposed to prevent. (Far superior results may be achieved through behavioral medicine by using a combination of **tryptophan loading** and **cognitive positivism**, techniques #5 and #17.

Yet another prophylactic drug prescribed for cluster headaches, lithium carbonate, poses a risk of kidney damage when employed for long-term use.

Among other drugs not to take for headaches are tranquilizers or muscle relaxants. Although they provide symptomatic relief of anxiety and tension, they intensify headache pain and often increase anxiety instead of relieving it.

Women may also want to avoid oral contraceptives. Roughly half of all women using the pill have complained of headaches after the first year. Powerful vasoconstrictors, oral contraceptives have been known to cause migraine accompanied by symptoms so severe that medical attention has been necessary. Headaches are also a common side effect of nitroglycerine and many other drugs.

This book will bring readers to the following conclusions:

1. Most drugs merely mask symptoms. Not a single drug can remove the underlying cause of most headaches, which is unresolved emotional stress.

2. Any therapy that does not use drugs offers enormous advantages over therapies that involve drug use.

ESCAPING THE DRUG TRAP

Assuming you are taking one or more OTC medications, which were not prescribed by a physician, the choice to stop using them is entirely up to you.

Before continuing to take any type of drug, you may want to ask yourself these questions:

Why am I taking this medication?

Is it really necessary and do I really need it?

What would happen if I did not take it?

What alternative therapies might be more effective, less costly, and free of destructive side effects? For example, before continuing to take a tranquilizer, have you considered such alternatives as exercise, deep breathing or deep relaxation—all much more effective, safer and cheaper than any drug?

These questions are not intended to discourage you from seeing a doctor, or from taking any drug that is really necessary. Obviously, some people are entirely unsuited to any form of therapy but drugs.

The idea is to get you thinking about stopping any drug that is not really needed. It is essential to try to minimize intake of every type of drug, because drugs may inhibit the effectiveness of natural therapies. Again, if you are taking a drug, it is difficult to assess the effects of behavioral medicine.

Meanwhile, if you must take drugs:

• Always take as few as possible.

• Ask for the minimum effective dosage for the shortest period of time.

BEAT HEADACHE MISERY WITHOUT USING DRUGS

Doctors are under tremendous pressure by drug manufacturers to place as many people as possible on lifelong maintenance drugs. All too often, both doctors and patients fail to realize that long-term use of headache drugs can lead to helplessness, hopelessness, depression and anxiety. In turn, these negative emotions merely exacerbate headache pain.

In reality, virtually all the functions achieved by drugs can also be achieved by using natural, drugless therapies instead. For example, drugs attempt to stop headache pain by intervening in bodily processes that are normally controlled by the involuntary nervous system. Most doctors consider that anything controlled by the involuntary nervous system is beyond our personal control. But behavioral medicine has effectively smashed this cherished belief by demonstrating that we can gain indirect control of several of the most important body functions involved in the headache process. In some cases, the techniques in this book may seem so indirect that it is like putting on a wool hat to warm the feet (actually one of the most effective ways to keep the feet warm). In headache therapy, by warming the hands and feet, we can draw blood away from the head and forestall a migraine attack.

CONTROL YOUR HEADACHE WITH NATURAL THERAPIES

It may be difficult at first to see that by creating an upbeat attitude, Chapters 2 and 3 actually put you in direct control of your headache. As you are transformed from a passive headache victim to a confident, medically-informed layperson, any tendencies toward helplessness, hopelessness, depression or anxiety should swiftly fade away. You learn that drugs are not the only way to overcome headaches and you become motivated to take an active role in your own recovery.

In Chapter 5, you learn to control foods that may be triggering your headache. You learn how to control low blood sugar. You learn how to control the migraine process with vitamins and minerals. And you learn how to control an important painkilling neurotransmitter in the brain by manipulating certain foods.

Chapter 6 reveals how to control headaches with a painkilling herb available in most health food stores, and how to control your headache through homeopathy.

Chapter 7 is filled with natural therapies that give you control over the diameter of your arteries and over defusing stress, anxiety and depression. You also learn how to control release of the brain's natural morphine-containing opiates that block headache pain from being experienced.

There are breathing techniques that can stop a migraine or cluster headache within minutes. And easy stretching techniques put you in control of chronic tension headaches.

In Chapter 8 you learn to use relaxation and biofeedback to gain control of your own involuntary nervous system. Through creative imagery you also learn how to mobilize your own body's placebo effect. Research has shown that, through the placebo effect, people with a strongly positive attitude recover 25–33 percent faster from *any* kind of ailment, disease or dysfunction from a minor headache to major surgery.

Again, through positivism, Chapter 9 helps you to gain direct control over your negative beliefs, thoughts and emotions—the underlying causes of almost all headaches. By controlling your thoughts, you can control your feelings—and can work toward feeling terrific all of the time.

Finally, Chapter 10 shows you how to take direct control of your life by helping you build a headache-free lifestyle.

FINDING YOUR WAY OUT OF THE DRUG JUNGLE

The trouble with relying on drugs to relieve headache pain is that their painkilling effect steadily loses power, forcing the sufferer to take ever-stronger painkillers with increasingly potent side effects. As these new, stronger drugs also continue to lose effectiveness, chronic headache victims are typically shuttled from one specialist to another, none of whom can find anything wrong. All too often, they are finally told by their own doctor, "There is nothing more that modern medicine can do. You'll just have to learn to live with your headache."

By showing that there are, indeed, many things that can be done to relieve headache pain, behavioral medicine offers new hope and optimism to all who are trying to find their way out of the drug jungle.

A cautionary note: While these natural therapies have been used with considerable success by a number of headache and pain clinics, there is, of course, no guarantee that any one therapy is going to work for everyone, or in every case every time. All we can say is that these methods have been reported to be successful at least 50 percent of the time. Naturally, if a therapy does not appear to work for you, you should switch to another alternative healing modality.

2 When to Seek Medical Help For Your Headache

Every year, tens of thousands of Americans mistakenly believe that their headache is due to a brain tumor or other serious disease. Records show that when this possibility is ruled out, almost every patient shows a significant and immediate improvement.

Anxiety worsens all headaches. By obtaining medical assurance that your headache is benign, you can work wonders in lessening anxiety. The relief that this news brings is often the biggest single step toward headache recovery. Furthermore, those who visit a headache or pain clinic are often delighted to learn that they can improve their condition while, at the same time, being weaned from drugs.

OBTAINING MEDICAL ASSURANCE THAT YOUR HEADACHE IS BENIGN

The remainder of this chapter covers how to go about seeking medical evaluation and the best ways to obtain it.

All headaches fall into one of two classes: disease-related or benign. The natural drugless therapies in this book are for use exclusively with benign headaches. So before reading on, it's important to make absolutely *certain* that your headaches really are benign. If your headaches are disease-related, you must seek medical advice and you should refrain from using any of the techniques in this book unless you have your physician's specific approval.

If you have been experiencing tension or migraine headaches for years, and the symptoms are not worsening, there probably isn't any urgent need for a medical checkup. A thorough evaluation by a headache clinic may cost $250–$500, and may be unnecessary for most people who suffer from a well-established pattern of chronic headaches. Only if symptoms are worsening, or if the pain is becoming unbearable and interfering with your work or family or social life, would you normally need to think about consulting a headache clinic.

Most of the therapies described in this book are similar or identical to those used by the majority of headache clinics. However, if you have any reason to think that you may require medical treatment, you should see your doctor or arrange to visit a headache clinic without delay.

Likewise, if you have any anxiety about your health and your headaches, you should arrange for a medical examination. Preferably this should be at a headache clinic. Or failing that, at a pain clinic or by a doctor who is experienced in headaches.

CHOOSING A HEADACHE OR PAIN CLINIC

Approximately 25 headache clinics exist in the U.S. The best are usually branches of major medical centers or universities, offer a multi-disciplinary (Whole Person) approach, and are staffed by specialists representing an array of disciplines, such as internists, neurologists, psychiatrists, physical therapists, and counselors. Other clinics may be operated by individual doctors with varying capabilities. It's best to seek a certified facility.

While most can be depended on for an expert diagnosis, smaller clinics may not offer the same wide option of alternative therapies as large, multi-disciplinary clinics. To help evaluate a clinic, check on the credentials of the staff and ask to see if they are board-certified in their field.

Most of America's several hundred pain clinics are also capable of diagnosing headaches, but not all specialize in headache treatment. Although the clinic itself may offer a multidisciplinary approach to pain relief, the headache department may offer only a single discipline. By comparison, virtually all bona fide headache clinics prefer a nondrug approach with emphasis on relaxation and biofeedback training, nutrition, massage, counseling and stress management. While some clinics accept patients without referral, others may require that you be referred by your doctor.

The average physician is probably quite capable of determining whether your headaches are disease-related or benign, but may not be as adept at diagnosing your headache *type*, and so may prescribe an inappropriate medication. The average doctor is also often unaware of the alternative, nondrug therapies used by most headache clinics, and will tend to rely upon drugs.

It is fairly common, in fact, for headache clinics to discover a misdiagnosis by a family doctor, who has also prescribed the wrong medication. When the medication is corrected and the patient introduced to other therapies, some patients are able to end their headaches in a short time.

How long does it normally take for a headache clinic to end chronic headaches permanently? That depends. In very stubborn cases, clinics may only be able to reduce the pain to manageable levels.

By contrast, benign chronic headaches can occasionally be permanently ended by a single therapy. But it's safest not to expect a magic bullet. Most clinics employ a holistic array of therapies that work on body, mind and belief system simultaneously. By working together synergistically, each reinforcing the other, a selection of these therapies can typically be expected to eliminate chronic migraine headaches in from 5 to 12 weeks.

WHEN SHOULD YOU SEEK MEDICAL HELP FOR YOUR HEADACHE?

If you have any of the following symptoms, seek medical care *immediately*. If circumstances warrant, call an ambulance or have someone take you to the nearest hospital emergency room.

A headache associated with loss of movement on one side of the body.

A new, sharp, sudden, severe or stabbing headache that causes you to stop whatever you're doing.

A headache in which it is painful to bend the head forward and which may also be accompanied by fever, drowsiness, altered moods, nausea or light hurting the eyes.

A very severe headache that is new or unusual.

Any headache that occurs after a recent head or neck injury.

Any headache accompanied by dizziness, double vision or loss of memory.

Any headache that makes you feel ill, especially if you have difficulty finding the right words or in calculating.

You're over 50 and have a headache associated with

fever, eyesight problems, weight loss and a pain on one side of the jaw while chewing.

You have a sudden, explosive, thunderclap-type headache for the first time, especially if it is the worst headache of your life.

Your headache is associated with fever, convulsions or loss of consciousness.

Symptoms such as these could indicate such serious disorders as a ruptured aneurysm or a blood clot in a carotid or inter-cranial artery, a stroke, meningitis, a brain tumor, an epileptic seizure or temporal arteritis.

Brain tumors are actually quite rare and you are very unlikely to have one. A brain tumor headache becomes progressively worse, and is accompanied by vomiting and severe disturbances of vision, speech or personality. Even then, many cases can be treated by surgery or radiation.

While the following headache symptoms don't require *immediate* attention, you should see a doctor as soon as possible.

You're over 50 and have a headache for the first time.

A young child has a persistently recurring headache.

Your headache symptoms differ from preceding patterns, especially if associated with pain in an eye or ear.

A headache is frequent, severe and sudden.

A headache occurs almost daily.

A headache occurs during or immediately after exercise, lovemaking or a bowel movement; or when coughing, bending, straining or sneezing.

A headache begins when you wake up from a sound sleep.

A headache is so severe that you must take pain relievers daily or almost daily.

You experience any sudden deteriorating change in headache pattern.

You have a headache that grows progressively severe as time goes on and is always in the same location.

A headache lasts 12 hours or more without dissipating.

A headache is accompanied by numbness in an arm or leg.

You have always experienced migraine pain on one side of the head and now it shifts to the other side.

For the first time you have a headache accompanied by visual disturbances, or weakness of one side of a body area, or dizziness or speech disorders.

A headache recurs in a similar pattern day after day, under the same circumstances, at the same time, in the same location, and for the same duration.

A headache is new and persistent when previously you had no headaches.

A headache is persistent and incapacitating.

A headache cannot be numbed by the strongest over-the-counter medications.

While such symptoms could be less urgent indicators of the same disorders described earlier, they could also be due to infections such as the Epstein-Barr virus. Requiring less urgent medical treatment are headaches due to a sinus infection, eyestrain, a deviated septum or hypertension.

ALMOST ALL HEADACHES ARE BENIGN

The message of this chapter is that if you have symptoms of any disease-related headache, you should consult a physician or headache clinic. Only after you have been assured that your headache is benign should you practice any of the therapies in this book. And for that also, you are advised to consult a doctor first.

The symptoms for disease-related headaches described in this chapter apply to fewer than two percent of all headaches. Which means that more than 98 percent of all headaches are benign. Although painful and, at times, even debilitating, a benign headache is not due to any underlying disease or disorder. Nor will it directly pose a threat to your health.

These caveats dispensed with, the remainder of this book is about benign headaches, and how you can help prevent and overcome these disorders without resorting to either OTC or prescription drugs.

3 Understanding Headache Dynamics Is the Key to Relief

The more you learn about the basics of headache mechanisms, the less reason you have to fear headaches. A sound knowledge of the headache process can give you a powerful feeling of being in control of not only your headache but of your health and life as well.

No longer do you need to feel a victim of random attacks . . . or totally dependent on drugs.

GAINING POWER OVER YOUR HEADACHE BY BECOMING MEDICALLY INFORMED

Choosing to learn more about the headache process is the first step in using behavioral medicine, the medical extension of holistic healing. By simply understanding how your body-mind produces a headache, you will find yourself transformed from a passive, helpless headache victim into a confident, medically informed layperson ready to take an active role in overcoming your chronic headache.

Before you can intervene successfully in your headache, you must know which type of headache you have. Basically, there are two types, disease-related headaches and benign recurrent headaches.

Disease-related headaches were discussed in Chapter 2. If you have not already done so, you should read Chapter 2 now. Disease-related headaches may require immediate medical attention. The natural therapies in this book are *not* intended for people with disease-related headaches.

All other headaches are classified as benign.

Benign Recurrent Headaches

Two types of benign headaches exist: Muscle Contraction Headaches and Vascular Headaches.

Muscle Contraction or Tension Headaches account for the vast majority of headaches. Almost invariably they are caused by unresolved emotional stress which is translated through the fight-or-flight response into abnormal contraction of the shoulder, neck and scalp muscles. There are two classes of tension headaches.

Acute tension headaches are isolated headaches generally caused by stress. They can normally be relieved by OTC drugs or by natural therapies and medical help is seldom required.

Chronic tension headaches persist day after day without relief. Many chronic tension headaches are linked to anxiety and depression and can continue without letup for years. Drugs serve only to temporarily relieve symptoms. The only treatment that really works is **Cognitive Positivism** (Technique #17).

Some variants of tension headaches are combination tension-vascular headaches, including exertion headaches, and those associated with temporomandibular joint syndrome, or TMJ. These are discussed after the next section, on vascular headaches.

Vascular Headaches. Usually caused by unresolved emotional stress, which triggers the fight-or-flight response, these headaches are set in motion by a complex series of biochemical reactions that cause changes in blood vessels and in blood flow in the head.

Whether or not the fight-or-flight response sets off a muscle contraction headache, or a vascular headache, or no headache at all, appears to depend on an individual's personal neurological chemistry. Headache specialists prefer to say that one person may have a biochemical predisposition to tension headaches, for example, while another may have a predisposition to migraine headaches. In either case, the headache mechanism is set in motion when the fight-or-flight response is invoked.

The most common vascular headache is migraine, which has several variants: some exertion headaches; hangover; caffeine withdrawal; ice cream; hunger; and menstrual headaches. Cluster headaches are another type of vascular headache.

Migraine Headaches. There are two distinct types of migraine headaches.

Classic Migraine Headache in which the headache is preceded by a spectacular "aura," consisting of visual disturbances and distortions of senses and perceptions. Usually, these symptoms last from 10–30 minutes, sometimes up to one hour, before they fade away and the headache begins.

Only 20 percent of migraines are classic; the remainder are common migraines.

Common Migraine Headache in which the prodromal (aura) sensations are so diffuse that they often amount to no more than a vague feeling of fogginess and irritability. As these uncertain symptoms disappear, the severe throbbing pain of migraine begins.

Cluster Headaches. The other type of vascular headache is the dreaded cluster. Two different types of clusters have been identified.

- Episodic or Cyclic Cluster Headache recurs in a pattern. Four of every five cluster headaches are episodic. They usually occur in bouts (hence the name cluster), after which they disappear for a year or more before returning in another bout. Breathing pure oxygen can shorten 70 percent of cluster headaches 70 percent of the time. But it is inconvenient to carry an oxygen bottle around.

- Chronic Cluster Headaches are acute attacks that recur regularly without remission for a period of one year or more. They are difficult to prevent pharmaceutically and, though they can be treated with analgesics, the attack is often over before the painkiller has begun to work.

COMBINATION AND VARIANT HEADACHES

Approximately ten percent of people with chronic tension headaches experience an occasional migraine headache superimposed on the tension headache. At this time, their headache worsens and they feel the throbbing pain of a vascular headache in addition to the steady, dull ache of the tension headache.

This is believed to be due to a vascular component in

some tension headaches. Most combination headaches are free of aura displays but the symptoms of common migraine are superimposed on those of the tension headache. Such headaches are best treated as migraines until the migraine ends, at which time therapy should be resumed for the tension headache.

Sexual Headaches. Another combination variant is the Benign Sexual Headache. The headache appears in two ways: either as a steady ache starting a few minutes before orgasm; or as a pulsating headache that suddenly begins at or near climax. Either type of headache may persist for several hours.

Headache specialists have suggested that sexual headaches are due to a combination of muscle contraction and blood vessel dilation set off by a sudden increase in blood pressure resulting from the excitement and exertion. These headaches usually appear in middle-aged men who are overweight, sedentary and mildly hypertensive. After several months, they often disappear. Though physically harmless, a benign sexual headache can have a traumatic effect on a person's love life.

Since a sexual headache could be confused with a stroke, you should consult a physician to confirm that the headache is actually benign. Your doctor may suggest a combination of exercise coupled with gradual weight loss to effectively lower blood pressure and overcome the headache.

TMJ Headaches. A fairly common variant of tension headache is due to the TMJ or Temporomandibular Joint Syndrome. People with deep anxiety often grind their teeth while asleep. This creates a painful spasm in face, neck and jaw muscles, particularly in the temporomandibular joint at the hinge of the jaw. Nerves refer the pain up to the forehead where it manifests as a headache in the temples and behind or below the eyes. A sign that a headache may be due to the TMJ syndrome is tenseness in the jaw on awakening and a feeling that the teeth have been tightly clenched.

The TMJ syndrome can often be relieved through relaxation or biofeedback training (Chapter 8). Otherwise, one should consult a dentist, preferably a member of the American Association of Oral and Maxillofacial Surgeons. Dentists are generally more aware of the TMJ process than doctors, and most are equipped to solve the problem.

They do so by making a light acrylic splint to be worn between the teeth while asleep. By making the teeth mesh correctly, the splint relaxes the jaw muscles so that they remain unstressed throughout the night. This usually stops the headaches.

Menstrual Migraines. In diagnosing a benign headache, it is helpful to know that both tension and migraine headaches are twice as common in women as men. By comparison, 19 of every 20 cluster headache sufferers are male.

Seventy percent of migraine sufferers are women in their childbearing years. In 60 percent of women migraineurs, the attacks occur during the week preceding, or during, menstruation. Other women experience migraine at the midpoint of the menstrual cycle, during ovulation. Migraines related to the menstrual cycle are often called menstrual migraines.

Menstrual migraines usually end by the third month of pregnancy, and the arrival of menopause liberates most women from further migraines. These clues indicate that migraine is related to hormone instability. And, indeed, taking estrogen or birth control pills *can* increase the frequency and intensity of migraine in women.

Most headache specialists believe that migraines are due to an inherited biochemical or hormonal imbalance. As a result, migraines tend to run in families. Thus children may experience migraines at a quite early age. Symptoms are similar to those in adults. Any child with migraine should be checked by a pediatrician to rule out the possibility of a disease-related headache.

Efforts to define a migraine personality have been unsuccessful, but many migraineurs seem to have low blood pressure, flexible arteries, cold hands, low blood sugar and unusually sensitive nerves. Women may experience menstrual irregularities. Classic migraineurs tend to be perfectionists, compulsively tidy and well-groomed, and may speak in hurried phrases. Many high achievers have been migraine sufferers.

Our personal observations indicate that the majority of people who suffer chronic headaches, both tension and migraine, are unable to handle stress in a relaxed way. Perhaps this is one reason why headaches are more common in younger than in older people. Headaches are most prevalent in women aged 20 to 30 and in men aged 30 to 40.

UNLOCKING THE SECRETS OF HEADACHE PATHOLOGY

Until recently, it was thought that headaches were caused by muscle contraction or by changes in blood vessels. Now we know that these phenomena are merely part of a deeper and more complex biochemical and neurological process. There is also a growing recognition that the underlying cause of nearly all benign headaches is unresolved emotional stress.

We have now learned that most headaches develop in four separate stages, and that each stage has its specific treatment requirements, whether by drugs or by behavioral medicine. Drugs or natural therapies that work in Stage 2, for example, are often not effective in Stages 3 or 4; and *only* nondrug therapies are effective in Stage 1.

By learning about these stages, you can easily recognize

the stage which your headache has reached. You can then choose the most appropriate anti-headache technique for that stage.

STAGE 1

Stage 1 is common to all three types of headaches: tension, migraine and cluster headaches.

New information emerging from the research frontiers of medical science is revealing that the underlying cause of most chronic, recurrent headaches is chronic, recurrent stress. As previously explained in Chapter 1, at least 80 percent of all headaches are believed to be set off by unresolved emotional stress.

Our lives today are filled with potentially stressful events capable of triggering a painful headache. Conflicts concerning job, family, money and relationships; noise and constantly ringing telephones; traffic jams and waiting in line, long tiring drives on the freeway . . . the modern world is filled with potentially headache-provoking situations.

However, stress is caused by the way we react to a situation, not by the situation itself. Most migraine sufferers characteristically overreact to events they perceive as immediately threatening or disturbing, while most tension headache sufferers tend to be anxious and worried about upcoming events.

We can understand how headaches begin when we realize that every feeling (emotion) is preceded by a thought. Whenever we think a positive thought, we experience a positive emotion such as love, joy, hope, compassion, contentment or gratitude. Whenever we think a negative thought, we swiftly experience a negative emotion such as fear, anger, hostility, resentment, guilt, frustration, envy or anxiety.

Positive thoughts arise from positive beliefs held in our

belief system while most negative thoughts arise because we continue to hold outdated conditioned beliefs that we acquired in the past and that are no longer valid or appropriate.

The human mind has been aptly described as a biological computer. Information about the world around us is fed into the brain's interpretive center, where it is matched with data held in our belief system. After perceiving the input data through a filter of our beliefs, our interpretive center responds by placing a thought in our mind.

For example, if we have just learned that a friend has been given a promotion that we expected to get, this information is matched in our belief system with associations from the past. Depending on the beliefs in our data banks, our mind could choose a positive, loving thought that makes us feel glad for our friend's success. Or it could choose the negative thought that considering all the hard work we'd put in over the years without recognition, *we* should have been chosen for the promotion instead.

If a positive thought arose, it would immediately provoke a positive feeling. And a negative thought would provoke a negative feeling. We experience our feelings in the limbic area of the brain that surrounds the hypothalamus and pituitary glands. These glands scan every feeling we experience.

The Healing Power of Positive Beliefs

Positive emotions are recognized as friendly, which is a signal for the glands to turn on the body's relaxation response. This is a calm, relaxed state of serenity and peace. The parasympathetic branch of the autonomic nervous system takes over and maintains routine metabolism. Muscular tension melts away and negative thoughts and feelings disappear. The heart rate drops, blood pressure falls, respiration slows, oxygen consumption is reduced and immunocompetence soars.

As we enter the relaxed alpha state, brainwave frequency drops to 8 to 13 cycles per second. We feel comfortable and relaxed and we experience a delightful state of ease and wellness in which headaches are rarely experienced.

By contrast, the hypothalamus and pituitary glands recognize all negative emotions as threatening or unfriendly. Whenever confronted with a negative feeling, even a mildly negative feeling like boredom or uncertainty, these twin glands turn on all or part of the body's fight-or-flight response.

Negative Beliefs as a Cause of Headache

Fight-or-flight is a hair-trigger response that evolved in primitive times to prepare the body to meet imminent physical danger. The sympathetic nervous system, the emergency branch of the autonomous nervous system, takes over and all systems are Go. The adrenal glands squirt hormones into the blood stream to speed up body functions. Nerve fibers signal the smooth muscles to constrict every artery and arteriole. Blood pressure shoots up, and blood is shunted from the digestive system to the brain and muscles. Glycogen (sugar) is released from the liver, filling our muscles with energy and tensing them for action. Meanwhile, the clotting ability of blood platelets increases in preparation for a possible wound.

The problem is that this response, a legacy from precaveman days, can be turned on by any kind of feeling that the hypothalamus and pituitary glands interpret as negative. All too many people have such inappropriate belief systems that a letter from the IRS can trigger the same emergency state that their ancestors would have experienced on being confronted by a saber-toothed tiger.

If we act out the fight-or-flight response by either fighting or fleeing (or by jogging, bicycling, briskly walking or doing pushups), we release the pent-up muscular tension and the other stress mechanisms swiftly fade away. But if, as is so often true in modern society, physical action is impossible, we remain tensed-up and uncomfortable and we live through the day in a state of distress.

Trying to repress a negative emotion, which means concealing or burying or denying our discomfort, only intensifies our stress. Many people live in a continuously low-level emergency state with all their stress mechanisms constantly simmering. It is these stress mechanisms—the release of adrenal hormones, tensing of muscles, and heightened clotting ability of the platelets—that set off the remaining stages in the headache process.

Psychological Origin of Physical Disorders

In Stage 1, our negative thoughts are translated into physiological states that can produce an ulcer, a heart attack, a stroke, an infection, cancer or a headache. In fact, medical science now recognizes that virtually every disease or dysfunction has a stress component. Which disorder we actually get depends on our genetic makeup. If our coronary arteries are prone to spasm, a stress mechanism can set off unstable angina and a heart attack. If we are prone to headaches, we may get a tension, a migraine, or a cluster headache. The type we get will be the one to which our body chemistry makes us most prone.

Although Stage 1 is the cause of most headaches, drugs or medical treatment can be of little help at this level. This emphasizes once again that most drugs merely serve to palliate symptoms while the root cause of disease may be eliminated by drugless behavioral medicine.

The most effective single step that most chronic headache sufferers can take is to let go of all beliefs that cause or intensify headaches and to replace them with new beliefs that minimize headaches and that engender high-level wellness.

One can only guess at how many millions of migraine headaches are suffered annually by people who continue to believe "I will never forgive so-and-so because of what he or she did to me." Such a destructive belief is a "hair trigger" which can set off a headache on the slightest provocation.

Meanwhile, we estimate, every year at least several thousand migraineurs achieve immediate and permanent liberation from their headaches when they learn to forgive everyone whom they believe may have harmed them.

Through behavioral medicine, we can eliminate most stress, and thereby end most headaches, by changing the way we perceive events, so that instead of seeing them as threatening, we see them as neutral or friendly. Chapter 9 describes how to absorb into your belief system all new beliefs that lessen headache pain, and to drop all those that intensify headache pain.

STAGE 2

In this intermediate stage, stress mechanisms cause changes to blood vessels and to blood flow in the head. In Stage 2, each headache type follows a separate path.

Tension Headaches

As energy pours into muscles throughout the body, tensing them for emergency action, the shoulders, neck, scalp and facial muscles also contract. The trapezius muscle, which connects the shoulder, neck and collarbone, may contract into a knot.

In the neck area, muscles, nerves and arteries are all closely packed. Prolonged tension in the muscles of shoulders and neck excites neural pathways that refer pain impulses up to the sweatband area for a second phase of muscular contraction.

These nerve impulses control the synthesis of prostaglandin, a hormonelike substance released by the immune system in response to stress. Prostaglandin immediately induces contraction in the smooth muscles of blood vessels in the headband area, as well as making nerve endings in these blood vessels exquisitely sensitive to pain.

Prostaglandin synthesis is an essential step in muscle contraction headaches. To a lesser extent it also occurs in the vascular headache process. When this step is blocked by intervention, tension headache pain cannot be perceived.

Nowhere is constriction more evident than in the occipital artery, which supplies a network of arterioles that radiate out behind the ears and into the headband area of the scalp. In a desperate attempt to bring in more blood and oxygen, these blood vessels burst into a vigorous dilation.

The overall effect is to dilate blood vessels in a wide band around the head that includes the temples, forehead and hatband area.

All is now ready for the headache to begin in Stage 3.

Classic Migraine

Roughly one-fifth of all migraine headaches are the classic type, meaning that they are preceded by a series of prodromal sensations, commonly known as an *aura*. Appearing before the eyes as a dazzling display of star bursts,

zigzag lines and patches of blackness, these visual disturbances are dreaded by most migraine sufferers. After 10 to
30 minutes, the aura activity ends and the migraine pain
hits.

Besides visual disturbances, aura symptoms may include
numbness in an arm or leg; a slurring of words or similar
speech impediment; acute sensitivity to glaring, flashing or
flickering light; bizarre changes in smell, taste, or touch;
cold hands; weakness or numbness in one side of the body;
tingling in legs, arms, hands or face; nasal congestion;
watery eyes and difficulty in focusing eyes; distorted perception; and restlessness or confusion.

Some migraine sufferers worry that prodromal visual
disturbances may be due to a detached retina. Very rarely
is this so. Moreover, some people experience aura symptoms without ever experiencing any migraine pain. This is
known as a migraine equivalent. Here again, the symptoms are often confused with those of a transient ischemic
attack which may herald a stroke. However, a true migraine equivalent is not associated with a stroke.

Aura symptoms are purely neurological in origin and are
set off by a "nerve storm" that slowly moves across the
brain from front to back. This phenomenon, discovered in
the 1980s by Jes Oleson and Martin Lauritzen, two University of Copenhagen researchers, explains the aura effect
in terms of a partial shut-down of cerebral blood circulation.

As the aura commences, the Danish researchers discovered, there is a 25 percent drop in blood flow at the back
of the brain. In a wavelike motion, this depression moves
from the back of the brain to the front. As it moves, it
activates the visual cortex and sets off neurological mechanisms that produce the aura effect in front of the eyes.

Although the wave motion is neurological and emanates
from the central nervous system, the reduced blood flow is
actually created by the opening of blood vessels called

shunts. These carotid shunts bypass incoming blood from the carotid arteries and carry it directly back into the veins.

Normally, blood from the carotid arteries flows into smaller vessels, arterioles, where it oxygenates cells in the brain, scalp and face. After unloading its oxygen, the blood returns through tiny venules into the veins. However, when the shunts open, they create a significant reduction in blood flow to scalp and brain.

At the same time, norepinephrine, released by the fight-or-flight-response, affects receptors on blood vessel walls in the brain and scalp, causing artery constriction. This artery constriction and the shunts seriously deplete blood flow to brain and scalp.

This sets the stage for a rebound effect. In a sudden response to the shortage of oxygen, the blood vessels overdilate. The aura ends and conditions are ready for the migraine to begin.

Common Migraine

During stress-free periods, the adrenals secrete cortisol and other hormones which affect receptors on blood vessel walls, keeping arteries mildly constricted and preventing vasodilation. Output of these hormones wanes during evening hours and at night, and they reach their lowest level at around 3 or 4 A.M. The lower the level of these hormones, the greater the tendency of blood vessels to dilate, making vessels most likely to dilate in late evening or at night. Several hours after these low levels are experienced is the time when most migraines are apt to begin.

Whenever the fight-or-flight response is invoked, the neurotransmitter norepinephrine is released, causing platelets to clump. Platelets are disk-shaped structures in the bloodstream that can coagulate and cause a blood clot. They are also carriers of another neurotransmitter, serotonin. As norepinephrine is released in response to stress, the platelets clump and release serotonin.

Norepinephrine and serotonin are powerful vasoconstrictors but have little else in common. Norepinephrine is an excitatory stimulant that keeps the brain aroused and alert, while serotonin is a natural tranquilizer which functions by inhibiting nerve impulses. Between them, norepinephrine and serotonin work in tandem to control the body's pain process. A deficiency of norepinephrine can cause depression, while a deficiency of serotonin lowers the pain threshold.

THE MECHANICS OF MIGRAINE

Amino acids (proteins) in the foods we eat are the body's only source of norepinephrine and serotonin. The amino acid phenylalanine is the precursor of norepinephrine while tryptophan is the precursor of serotonin. Chronic migraine headache sufferers invariably have a deficiency of one or both.

Immediately the fight-or-flight response is evoked, norepinephrine is released. Swiftly it locks into beta receptors on blood vessels in the head, causing them to constrict powerfully. A few minutes later (typically 4 to 8 minutes), serotonin appears and intensifies the constriction, causing the blood vessels to go into spasm. Artery spasm is further enhanced by the presence of calcium. In vascular headaches, calcium must be present for arteries to constrict.

At this point, the immune system steps in and releases yet another chemical messenger, histamine, which creates inflammation by causing blood vessels to swell.

Both calcium and histamine must be present for the headache process to continue. If either is blocked by intervention, constriction ceases, artery walls return to normal size, and the headache is aborted. Not surprisingly, several anti-headache medications work by blocking one or other of these chemicals.

Next, serotonin teams up with a substance called brady-kinin. Together, they coat the arteries of scalp and brain, making these blood vessels extremely sensitive to pain. Blood flow to cells in the brain and scalp is then reduced.

Faced with this potent array of biochemicals, the stabilizing influence of the body's normal adrenohormone supply is powerless to prevent a rebound effect. In a desperate attempt to bring in more blood and oxygen, the blood vessels rebel with a sudden and explosive dilation.

Cluster Headaches

While emotional stress is often the underlying cause of cluster headaches, Stage 2 occurs without any sensations. Research has yet to uncover all the mechanisms involved in the cluster process. But several experts have suggested that stress hormones released in Stage 1 cause calcium to flow into the muscular walls of blood vessels in the brain and scalp.

The presence of calcium causes blood vessels to go into spasm and constrict. When cerebral blood vessels spasm, the biochemical histamine is released. Studies have shown that levels of histamine are sharply higher at the onset of a cluster headache while levels of other biochemicals, such as serotonin, remain constant.

STAGE 3

This is the dilation phase of the headache process. In all three headache types, actual pain occurs as arteries in the forehead, scalp and brain dilate. Fine nerve filaments (nerve plexuses), which line the walls of these arteries, are extremely sensitive to being stretched. When the arteries swell and distend, these nerves fairly scream with pain.

At no time does the brain itself experience pain, for it contains no sensory nerves. All intracranial sensitivity exists in the membranes, or meninges, that line the inner wall of the skull.

Tension Headache

Most tension headaches occur as arteries in the forehead, scalp and brain dilate. Other pain signals may be generated by nerve endings located in the contracted muscles of shoulders, neck and scalp. Several hours after the headache begins, these muscles begin to relax and cease to generate further pain signals. But it may be 12 hours before the headband arteries return to normal size and the headache dissipates spontaneously. Throughout the tension headache, blood flow to the head remains constant and unchanged.

Migraine Headaches

Although observations at headache clinics indicate that common migraine may be more painful than the classic variety, from the beginning of Stage 3 on, the headache process is virtually identical for both migraine types.

Once the cerebral blood vessels dilate, the headache begins. Occasionally, the pain is mild and bearable; more often it appears as a throbbing, hammering pain that envelops the eye and nostril on one side of the head.

The pain can become so severe that victims are unable to walk straight, and may bump into furniture. During some attacks, the pain is so disabling that the person becomes incapable of coherent thought. Roughly half of all migraineurs experience nausea and vomiting. Others are plagued by diarrhea, dizziness, or bouts of hot flashes alternated with shivering spells. It is not unusual to see the arteries pulsating on the scalp while veins on the forehead are also visibly swollen.

The pain may reach back and follow the temporal artery up and over the ear and back to the neck on the afflicted side. Rarely does migraine appear on both sides of the head at once. Gradually, what feels like army boots pounding on the skull gives way to a steady ache. The torment can last from three hours to three days.

Yet in most cases, the headache lasts only until the victim falls asleep. When the migraineur wakes up, the headache is gone. The sufferer may feel weak and washed out and may pass copious amounts of pale urine, but permanent physical damage is rare.

Migraine does not usually return until the supply of norepinephrine has been replenished. This normally guarantees freedom from another attack for at least several days.

MIGRAINE TRIGGERS

Whenever conditions conspire—stress mechanisms are simmering and adrenal hormone output is low—migraine can be triggered by a food or environmental stimulant. During evening and early night hours, almost anything with vasodilatory powers can set off neurological mechanisms that dilate blood vessels in the head.

Among the most common vasodilating foods and beverages are aged wines, alcohol, some beers, yogurt, pickles, cheeses, caviar, pickled herring, cured meats, liver, monosodium glutamate, hot dogs, milk, meat, eggs and soy products. Many of these foods contain vasodilators such as nitrites, tyramine or phenylalanine.

Other common migraine triggers include

skipping meals

low blood sugar or hunger

strenuous physical exertion

ice cream or other cold foods
or drinks

high altitude

flickering lights or bright,
glaring sunlight

hot, dry winds or weather

smog and sulphur dioxide
emissions from industrial
plants

smoking

pollen and dust

wearing swim goggles or
mask

loud noise

oral contraceptives

excitement

abrupt changes of posture

some medications, especially
nitroglycerine (a potent
vasodilator)

premenstrual period

ICE CREAM AND HANGOVER HEADACHES

Fortunately, most migraineurs are sensitive only to one or two of these triggers. But cold can be a trigger for one migraineur in three. These people experience a sharp pain in the forehead or temple after swallowing ice cream or an iced drink. Often called the "ice cream headache," it is believed to be caused by irritation to nerve endings in the mouth or face. Pain impulses are referred by the trigeminal nerve to the forehead area where they set off blood vessel dilation and create a vascular headache. Exposure to icy winds or to any kind of cold on the face, or to diving into cold water, can also excite nerves that set off a migrainelike pain in the forehead or temple.

Yet another vascular variant is the hangover headache, caused by overindulgence in alcohol, a powerful stimulant that dilates arteries inside the skull so that bending forward increases the pain. In this same class are rebound headaches, due to withdrawal from vasoconstrictors such as caffeine, nicotine or ergotamine.

Cluster Headaches

Clusters are almost always limited to males 20 to 50 years of age. Many have a long history of excessive cigarette smoking and alcohol consumption. A combination of smoking, shallow breathing, a slouching posture, and lack of exercise results in a chronically low level of oxygen intake.

An immediate result of Stage 2 artery constriction is release of the biochemical histamine. The histamine immediately dilates the internal carotid artery. Surrounding this artery is a network of parasympathetic nerves that cause the eye and nose to relax. Pressure from the swollen carotid artery stimulates these nerves. In turn, the nerves dilate arteries in the eye and nose area.

The role of the parasympathetic nervous system is to turn on relaxation. Almost at once, the eye and nose begin to relax. The eyelid droops and the pupil contracts, while the nostril becomes congested on the afflicted side of the face. Meanwhile, blood flow to the face increases and the facial temperature rises. Simultaneously, in a last-ditch effort to restore oxygen levels, blood vessels in the scalp and brain commence a vigorous dilation.

The pain begins without warning and ceases without warning 10 to 30 minutes later. The headache develops around and behind one eye and may radiate to the forehead, temple or nose. The pain is usually on one side only and usually continues to occur on that same side.

THE AGONY OF CLUSTER HEADACHES

The pain is excruciating, boring into the eye and reaching such intensity that the victim becomes nauseated and vomits. On the affected side, the eye becomes red and swollen. The eyelid droops and the pupil contracts. The face becomes flushed and sweat may appear on the forehead. Vision may blur on the affected side. Frequently, the pain is so severe that the victim strides up and down, hand clasped over the painful eye. The pain can be so unbearable that the sufferer bangs his head against a wall or contemplates suicide.

While one headache a day is typical, some sufferers experience as many as three. In the episodic or cyclic type of cluster, the headaches occur only during a bout which typically lasts from two to eight weeks. After that, the headaches go into remission and do not reappear for months or even years. However, chronic clusters continue for a year or more without remission. Any severe one-sided headache involving changes to eyelid or pupil could well be a cluster.

WHO GETS CLUSTERS AND WHEN

The majority of clusters occur at night. Researchers believe that this may be due to a combination of shallow breathing and the daily low point in adrenal hormone output. (Normally, these hormones keep blood vessels from dilating.) These circumstances, which favor dilation, seem to set a regular time for clusters to appear. During a cluster bout, the victim is often awakened at the same time each night by the same blinding pain.

Whenever instability occurs in the balance of norepinephrine and serotonin, which control pain perception, clusters may also appear during the daytime. In fact, during a cluster bout, any food, substance or circumstance that stimulates vasodilation can trigger a cluster.

Clusters usually begin in men between the ages of 10 and 30, often in teenage boys who smoke. No family history connection has been found. Beyond causing a tendency to peptic ulcers, the pain appears to leave no lasting damage. But signs of suffering are often evident. By middle age, many cluster victims have acquired deep furrows in the forehead plus a cleft chin, square jaw and other craggy features, and a coarse, ruddy, wrinkled skin.

Fortunately, cluster headaches are relatively rare. At times, they may be confused with trigeminal neuralgia— tic douloureux. However, tic douloureux strikes in brief, painful jabs seldom lasting more than a few seconds, while clusters last for at least ten minutes.

Breathing pure oxygen is an effective remedy for most clusters at this stage. If oxygen is not available, hyper- ventilation—taking long, deep, rapid breaths—will often bring sufficient oxygen into the arteries to cause them to constrict and end the pain.

STAGE 4

In all three headache types, pain is actually perceived in the cortex of the brain. Electrochemical impulses gener- ated by tortured nerve endings in swollen head arteries carry the pain signal along neural pathways and through the spinal column into the midbrain and hypothalamus. The more rapid the impulses, the greater the intensity of pain registered in the brain.

In this stage, the pain process is approximately the same in all three headache types.

All Headache Types

Relayed from one nerve cell to the next by neurotrans- mitters, pain impulses from swollen head arteries travel along the triple-branched trigeminal nerve to the spinal cord. Once in the brain, all pain impulses are borne along by a neurotransmitter called Substance P.

In the dorsal horn of the spinal cord is a neurological "gate." Nerve messages from all over the body converge on this gate before entering the brain. Only a certain number of pain impulses can pass through the gate at one time. When other messages that seem more important are jamming the gate, pain impulses are unable to pass.

Most of us have experienced this phenomenon when we incurred a sports injury. So intent were we on winning or scoring that the pain went unnoticed until the game ended. At this point, messages about the game ceased and pain impulses were able to break through—and we knew we were hurting!

During World War II pain researcher Henry Beecher found that wounded soldiers required far less morphine than civilians with comparable injuries. He concluded that being injured was traumatic for a civilian, and produced great anxiety, while for a soldier, being injured brought relief at being taken out of battle.

Anxiety versus relief work in tandem to control entry of headache impulses through the pain gate. This translates biochemically into pain control by norepinephrine and serotonin, as they also work in tandem. Norepinephrine is produced through stress mechanisms turned on by anxiety and similar fear-based negative emotions. A high level of negative emotions produces a high level of norepinephrine, allowing an excessive number of pain impulses to pass through the gate.

Alternatively, positive emotions calm and relieve the mind so that additional serotonin from the diet can penetrate the blood-brain barrier and reach the brain. A sufficiency of serotonin restricts pain impulses from passing through the gate and also reduces perception to pain.

The Body's Own Natural Narcotics Deaden Pain

From the gate, pain impulses travel on to the midbrain. At work in both locations are two types of opiatelike brain chemicals, the smaller, shorter-acting enkephalins, and the longer-lasting endorphins. Acting like morphine, these substances can deactivate Substance P, stalling and blocking pain impulses.

These painkilling chemicals are also controlled by the delicate balance of norepinephrine and serotonin. A sufficiency of serotonin enhances the ability of endorphins to lock into anti-pain morphine receptors in the brain, thus effectively blocking pain impulses.

While norepinephrine and serotonin are released by the adrenal glands in response to stress, they are also produced in the brain. One way to ensure having sufficient serotonin is to eat enough foods containing tryptophan, serotonin's precursor. (See Technique #5.)

In this way, enkephalins and endorphins effectively control an individual's pain threshold. In chronic headache victims, endorphin levels are invariably low. This is because repeated stress totally consumes the endorphin supply, leaving one defenseless against pain. Abnormally low endorphin levels have also been found in other painful disorders known to develop from chronic stress.

Scientists have thus discovered the mechanism through which negative emotions such as anger, hostility, bitterness, or hopelessness, deplete the body's store of endorphins, seriously reducing a person's ability to tolerate pain.

The good news is that two natural therapies can swiftly replenish the endorphin supply. They are *rhythmic exercise* and *thinking positively*, so that we experience only positive emotions. Endorphin supplies can be boosted significantly by an hour of brisk exercise. As soon as it is released in the brain, endorphin begins to block pain receptors, creating a delicious pain-free high with upbeat feelings of sharpness and alertness. Positive thinking creates a similar upbeat state of pain-free consciousness.

The Limited Benefits of Headache Drugs

Based on a series of double-blind studies at leading university medical centers, approximately one-third of the beneficial effect of drugs comes not from any pharmaceutical action but from the body-mind's own placebo effect. The placebo effect stems from the patient's *belief* in a therapy rather than from the therapy itself.

Through the faith of believing in a medication or therapy, hope is aroused, and the mind begins to work independently of the treatment. It begins to harness the body's own natural healing powers. Among the principal healing forces mobilized by the placebo effect are endorphins and enkephalins. Through a combination of nondrug therapies—positive thinking and rhythmic exercise, for example—endorphin is often released in such amounts that these hormones can completely block severe headache pain.

A dramatic example of the placebo effect is seen when headache sufferers who believe they have a brain tumor are told by a physician that they do not. At least half of these patients show immediate and significant improvement. Their joy and relief releases clouds of endorphin that effectively block every pain receptor in the brain. As they experience this exhilarating feeling of pain-free ease, their mood soars into a euphoric state of high-level wellness. For many, this transformation from helplessness to joy is proof that they can overcome their chronic headaches without drugs.

Those pain impulses that survive the spinal cord gate and the activity of enkephalins and endorphins in the midbrain are relayed on through the hypothalamus and pituitary glands to the cortex, where pain perception actually occurs.

Here again, the extent of pain actually felt is controlled by the balance between norepinephrine and serotonin. Depletion of either can lead to depression. It hardly seems surprising then that chronic headache and depression so frequently occur together.

DEAR DIARY: A POWERFUL HEALING TOOL

Keeping a headache diary is standard practice at headache clinics. By noting the circumstances surrounding each episode, you can often detect the cause of your headaches. Note down such vital facts as the day of the week and the season; duration and frequency of attacks; time of day; and what you ate, drank, thought, did or felt prior to the headache. Are your headaches worsening or improving? Are you taking medications or oral contraceptives?

Was the pain steady or throbbing, confined to only one side of the head? Does it appear singly or in clusters? Does it occur during or after sex, or after caffeine, alcohol or smoking? Was it preceded by a conflict or a stressful situation, or by exercise, or did you have a stressful day at work? How is the headache related to your menstrual period? And so on.

After a few weeks, a pattern should emerge which can help you identify stressful situations, possible migraine triggers and potential vasodilators or vasoconstrictors that could be causing your headaches.

KNOWLEDGE IS POWER

Through acquiring familiarity with each step of the headache process, headaches need no longer appear mysterious or frightening, nor hold any power over us. We now know that by using drugless behavioral medicine we ourselves can intervene successfully on all four headache levels.

Although we've covered all the headache basics in this chapter, you will find still other helpful facts and information in the chapters that follow. Once you have read this book right through, you will be very informed about headaches.

ADDITIONAL FREE HEADACHE INFORMATION

Further information is available from these sources.

National Headache Foundation
5252 North Western Avenue
Chicago, Il. 60625
Phone 1-800-843-2256. Offers educational materials
on headaches and list of physician members and clinics.
Annual membership was recently $15.

American Association for the Study of Headache
PO Box 5136
San Clemente, CA 92672
Can help you locate a headache clinic.

4 How to Start Feeling Better Right Away

Suppose you're just coming down with a headache. Which Anti-Headache Techniques can you use right away to relieve your pain and to start feeling better?

To begin with, you must be able to identify your headache type and, in some cases, the stage that it is in. That's why we've placed this section this far on in the book. (We assume you have already read Chapters 1, 2 and 3.)

Once you're certain which type of headache you have— *and that it is benign*—you can begin using a variety of Anti-Headache Techniques for temporary relief. These fast-acting techniques are intended only as a stopgap measure to give you time to read this book right through.

To ensure being able to launch a truly holistic approach, the only one that will get rid of your headaches permanently, you must read and absorb this book right through to the end.

Listed below are the best techniques for speedy relief of each headache type. The page number of each technique is given in the table of contents in front of this book. Full instructions for using each technique are thus easily found. The abbreviation AHT in the listings below stands for Anti-Headache Technique.

Cluster Headaches

AHT #8-A: Giving the One-Two Punch to Cluster Headaches.

Migraine Headaches

AHT #7: The Li-Shou Method.
AHT #8: Walk Your Headache Away.
AHT #9: Breathe Away Migraines.
AHT #9-A: Rub Away Headache Pain.
AHT #10: Banish Headaches With This Facial Tone-Up.
AHT #10-A: Morphine For the Mind.
AHT #11: Brush and Massage Your Headache Away.
AHT #12: Temperature Therapy For Speedy Relief.
AHT #12-A: Using Cold to Kill a Headache.

Tension Headaches

AHT #7: The Li-Shou Method.
AHT #8: Walk Your Headache Away.
AHT #9-A: Rub Away Headache Pain.
AHT #10: Banish Headache Pain With This Facial Tone-Up.
AHT #10-A: Morphine for the Mind.
AHT #11: Brush and Massage Your Headache Away.
AHT #12: Temperature Therapy For Speedy Relief.
AHT #12-A: Using Cold to Kill a Headache.
AHT #13: Quick Relief for Tension Headaches.

Hunger or Hypoglycemia Headaches

AHT #3-A: A Proven Remedy for Hypoglycemia Headaches.

Hangover Headaches

AHT #1: Quick Relief for Hangover Headaches.

5 The Nutritional Approach

Myfanwy Jones, a 40-year old secretary in Cardiff, Wales, had suffered from recurring migraine attacks for over ten years. The headaches kept her away from work for several weeks each year.

Finally, she consulted a specialist at London's Charing Cross Hospital. After a thorough examination, the specialist sent Myfanwy home with instructions to completely eliminate from her diet the ten most common foods that experience had shown triggered migraine headaches.

These foods were

all wheat and corn products

chocolate

all whole milk products, especially aged or yellow cheeses

all meats, fish or vegetables that are processed, cured, smoked, aged, marinated, pickled, salted or fermented (including bacon, ham, hot dogs and all types of sausage)

citrus fruits

MSG (monosodium glutamate)

all alcohol, especially red wines

beef, pork and liver

seafood and shellfish

all fried foods and fats

Myfanwy was to replace these foods with any selection of fresh fruits and vegetables, tubers, seeds, and other types of whole grains, augmented occasionally with small helpings of non-fried chicken, turkey or fish.

Although Myfanwy had serious doubts that her headaches were caused by what she ate, she stayed faithfully with her new diet. When three months had gone by without a single migraine, her views began to change.

"I never thought that the same foods I'd been eating since childhood, and that my parents and grandparents had eaten all their lives, could be causing my headaches," she said in an interview.

After the three-months trial period was over, Myfanwy found that she could safely eat wheat, corn and citrus without getting a headache. It was primarily foods of animal origin—that is, foods high in amines—that seemed to trigger her migraines.

Myfanwy's was one of the many similar cases which, a short while later, prompted Dr. Ellen Grant of London's Charing Cross Hospital, to study the effects of various foods on 60 chronic migraine patients. Dr. Grant found that when the ten most common migraine trigger foods were eliminated, 50 of the 60 persons in the study became completely headache-free.

Dr. Grant's is one of several landmark studies made in recent years which indicate that, by changing what, when and how we eat, a sizeable proportion of migraine attacks could be prevented.

GUILTY FOODS

Most clinical ecologists (allergy doctors) believe that migraine may be triggered by addictive cravings for foods that contain amines. Amines are precursors of several neurotransmitters that cause the brain to secrete enkephalin and endorphins, morphine-like narcotic painkillers. Eating amine-rich foods creates a painless high that makes us feel good. We then develop an addiction to these foods. When we stop eating them, we experience withdrawal symptoms. So we give ourselves another fix by eating more of the foods we crave. Regardless of how much we eat, we continue to crave these foods.

The catch is that most foods high in amines are also powerful vasodilators. In conjunction with emotional stress, and when the body's adrenal-hormone supply is at a low point in its daily cycle, amines from foods can easily trigger a Stage 3 dilation and set off migraine in a susceptible person.

Among the most potent vasodilators in common foods are:

tyramine, found in most red wines, cheeses, liver, cured meats and chocolate

octapamine, found in citrus

phenylethylamine, found in chocolate and alcohol

monosodium glutamate, found in Chinese restaurant food and in many canned and processed foods

sodium nitrite (and sodium nitrate), found in many types of cured meats

All foods containing these substances are high on the list of suspected migraine trigger foods.

Some other common migraine trigger foods are:

canned figs

non-white vinegar

yeast products, including
  yeast breads

nuts; dried peas and beans

ice cream

white flour

white sugar

most canned, preserved and
  processed foods

commercial salad dressings

eggs

chocolate milk

syrup

most commercial baked goods,
  especially pies, brownies,
  doughnuts, cookies, cakes
  and candies

☐ Anti-Headache Technique #1: Quick Relief for Hangover Headaches

Alcohol is another powerful vasodilator capable of triggering both migraine and cluster headaches. In people not susceptible to either of these types, it can set off a less severe, but still painful, hangover headache.

Alcoholic beverages which contain esters, aldehydes and phenolic flavonoids, such as red wines, are ranked among those most likely to provoke a headache. If you must drink, vodka is least likely to provoke a headache, followed by white wines, brandy and gin. Another way to prevent an alcohol-induced headache is to eat before drinking and to continue to eat and snack along with your drinks.

When consumed, all forms of alcohol are carried in the bloodstream to the liver where they are broken down into carbon dioxide, fatty acids and carbohydrate. The carbon dioxide sets off vasodilation in arteries inside the skull. This can trigger a cluster or migraine headache in susceptible people. For instance, a recent British study found that red wines precipitated migraines in 9 of 11 patients who suspected they were sensitive to alcohol.

Yet for most of us, overindulgence in alcohol is more likely to provoke a typical hangover headache, a pulsating, vascular type of head pain often accompanied by nausea. It can begin as early as one hour after drinking begins. Some people get hangover headaches after only one or two drinks. Others must indulge in several drinks before provoking a hangover headache. Often, the headache appears on waking up the morning after. Not surprisingly, hangover headaches are most common on Sunday mornings.

Several home remedies will help to relieve hangover headaches. Coffee will constrict dilated arteries and help to ease the headache pain.

But the *very best* remedy is a bowl of strong broth. Failing this, drink a glass of fruit or tomato juice in which you have dissolved a tablespoon of honey.

☐ Anti-Headache Technique #1-A: Prevent Headaches by Avoiding This Food Additive

Anyone prone to migraine should also studiously avoid exposure to MSG, monosodium glutamate. This popular flavor enhancer can also provoke a headache in people *not* prone to migraine. It is liberally used by cooks in Chinese restaurants. If you must eat in these restaurants, try to avoid beginning the meal with wonton soup, a small bowl of which typically contains 2.5 grams of MSG. Endeavor instead to eat some bread first, or any other food free of MSG, so that you do not consume the MSG-laden course on an empty stomach. Another food that may be high in MSG is hydrolized vegetable protein. Many Chinese restaurants will now serve food without MSG if you ask; it's a good idea to do so.

An MSG headache is actually caused by free glutamic acid which stimulates taste receptors on the tongue. The headache begins 20 to 30 minutes after eating MSG and is experienced as an ache or throbbing pain over the temples, in the forehead area, and also in the cheeks and jaw. It is sometimes accompanied by a burning sensation in the chest and upper torso. In non-migraineurs, it usually disappears within an hour.

☐ Anti-Headache Technique #2: How to End Caffeine Rebound Headaches

Caffeine is a legal form of speed that can both constrict and dilate arteries, and can also cause a painful rebound headache. In moderate quantities, say two to three cups a day, coffee is a powerful vasoconstrictor. Yet in larger amounts, such as five or more cups per day, it becomes a potent vasodilator.

In moderate quantities, coffee will relieve certain vascular headaches by constricting already dilated arteries. But in larger amounts, it causes blood vessels to dilate. It can also cause a rebound headache.

A rebound headache occurs when a caffeine addict misses a fix and begins to experience withdrawal symptoms. The dilated arteries will constrict again as soon as another cup of coffee is consumed. And the coffee-withdrawal headache swiftly disappears. Unfortunately, migraine headaches do not respond as readily to coffee, though tension headaches occasionally do.

When suffering from rebound headaches provoked by caffeine, the solution is to gradually reduce intake of not only coffee but of tea, cocoa, cola drinks and any other caffeine-containing beverages or medications. Otherwise, it's best to keep coffee intake down to not more than two or three cups per day. Besides causing headaches, caffeine has been implicated in causing insomnia and restlessness and in heightening risk of heart disease and bladder cancer.

☐ Anti-Headache Technique #3: Finding the Nutritional Fuse That Sets Off Your Headache

Not every migraine attack is triggered by a food. We should never forget that food triggers migraine 1) only when a person is already under emotional stress, and 2) when the stabilizing effect of normal adrenal hormone output is at a low point in its daily cycle. What this means is that without our being aware of it, Stages 1 and 2 in the headache process could have already occurred.

But studies have shown that at least 25 to 30 per cent of migraineurs can benefit from diet and nutritional therapy, while the elimination of trigger foods could probably prevent migraine attacks in as many more. It often is not necessary to give up all of the trigger foods listed in this chapter so far. Only a few may actually be triggering your headaches.

Assuming you are suffering from fairly frequent chronic migraines, you should be able to identify your personal trigger foods by using an elimination diet. This involves a simple three-step process.

• Step 1. Begin an anti-migraine diet, eating only foods unlikely to trigger a headache. If after ten days, your migraines have ceased, this is a good indication that your headaches may be due to one or more trigger foods.

• Step 2. Make a list of those foods or beverages you crave the most and which you suspect could be precipitating your headaches.

• Step 3. Every two days, reintroduce a single suspect food into your diet. During a 48-hour period, eat several helpings, especially in the evening. If you get a headache, eliminate that food and return to your anti-migraine diet for another 4 days. Then introduce the next suspect food. And so on.

At this point, you are cautioned not to begin an elimination diet without your doctor's specific approval. However, provided you do not test more than four foods at one time (over a total of eight days of testing), there is little risk for a healthy person. If at any time while on the elimination diet or while testing foods, you experience any unusual symptoms, pain, digestive disorder or pronounced discomfort, stop the diet and return to your normal eating patterns immediately.

On the other hand, you don't need to give in too easily. Don't give up just because you crave a certain forbidden food, or because it's difficult to adjust to new eating patterns, or because of pressure from relatives or friends.

IMPLEMENTING THE ELIMINATION DIET

Step 1: Adopt an Anti-Migraine Diet.

A diet of anti-migraine foods provides us with the nutritional opposite of migraine trigger foods. Since it is usually foods of animal origin (including eggs and whole milk dairy products) that are high in amines and amino acids, the anti-migraine diet is basically vegetarian. In fact, thousands have ended their chronic migraines for good simply by becoming strict vegetarians.

Not only does animal protein promote migraine but so do the saturated fats found almost exclusively in animal foods. Saturated fats stimulate release of a prostaglandin that causes blood platelets to set off the chain reaction leading to Stage 2 of the headache process. Fats of all kinds also increase absorption of amines.

These facts emerged during a recent study by pain control researchers at Temple University in Philadelphia. They found that a near-vegetarian diet low in fats, animal protein and refined carbohydrates significantly helped reduce or eliminate migraine pain. Seventy-five percent of the diet consisted of complex carbohydrates (fresh fruits, vegetables and whole grains). Excluded from the diet were all fats and oils (especially butter, margarine, lard, saturated fats and shortening); all white flour, sugar and sweeteners; all whole milk dairy products; all nondairy creamers; and all nuts, olives, preserves, jellies, candies or frozen fruit juices with sugar added.

Other studies have revealed that the more a food is processed or preserved, the more likely it is to trigger migraine. It makes sense, therefore, to avoid any prepared or processed foods containing fats, oils, sugar or eggs. In their place, we should eat freshly prepared primary foods (meaning foods exactly as they exist in nature). We should carefully avoid any aged, pickled, fermented, cured, smoked or marinated foods as well as all breakfast cereals that contain anything other than whole grains. Salt should also be minimized because it stimulates the vagus nerve in the stomach through which headache-producing impulses can be relayed.

Among foods which have a history of almost never triggering migraines are

melons
brown rice
rice flour
puffed rice
all sugar-free cooked or dry
   whole-grain breakfast cereals
pure fruit juices
cooked fruits

cooked whole grains (except
   wheat and corn)
raw seeds
bran muffins
tapioca
homemade vegetable soups
mixed vegetable juices

Almost all cooked vegetables are safe, especially sweet potatoes and other tubers, asparagus, carrots, eggplant, beets, pumpkin, spinach, squash, broccoli, cauliflower, Brussels sprouts and tomatoes. Many of these are delicious when steamed or baked in a casserole or made into a soup or stew. Also permitted are small, occasional helpings of deep sea fish like cod or haddock, lamb, turkey and chicken without the skin. Bake, broil, steam or boil but do not fry and never serve with any oil, fat or sweetener.

Although most raw fruits and vegetables rank among the healthiest foods, occasional ones have been identified as potential migraine triggers that, in relatively rare cases, may provoke a headache in certain individuals. Unlikely as the possibility is, any raw fruit or vegetables identified as a migraine trigger should be avoided until it can be tested and safely reintroduced into your diet. Among raw fruits and vegetables occasionally identified as migraine triggers are citrus, tomatoes, bananas, avocadoes, plums and prunes; and peanuts, peas, and onions.

The anti-migraine diet should be followed for up to ten days, or for any lesser period sufficient to demonstrate whether or not your headaches are food-related. If your headaches continue as usual, they are very likely not caused by foods and you should return to your normal diet. If your headaches disappear, this is a strong indication that they are triggered by one or more foods you normally eat.

The following two steps gradually introduce back into your diet every food that does not actually cause a headache.

Step 2: Pinpoint the Foods You Crave the Most

Most of us can identify our food addictions by answering these six questions and naming each food we crave.

1. Which foods do you eat most of and most often?
2. Which foods do you eat at almost every meal?
3. When you don't get a certain food, do you experience a let-down feeling?
4. Do you feel uncomfortable if a certain food is not available at each meal?
5. Can you relieve this discomfort by eating a certain food?
6. When you eat this food, do you still feel hungry and crave more of it?

Most people have fewer than a dozen foods which they actually crave. Make a list of these foods in the order in which you crave them most. By way of example, let's say that the foods on your list are: yellow cheeses; ice cream; chocolate; corn and corn products; pickled herring; bacon, ham; hot dogs; liver and beef.

Step 3: Identifying Your Personal Migraine Trigger Foods

Let's assume that after following the anti-migraine diet for up to ten days, your headaches have ceased. At this point, beginning with breakfast, you should begin to test the suspect food at the top of your list; we'll use yellow cheese as an example.

You do this by continuing to eat your anti-migraine diet. But at each meal, reduce your usual serving by about 15 per cent. In its place, add a fairly generous serving of yellow cheese. The later in the day, the larger you can make the helping of suspect food. However, do not eat more of the suspect food than you would in your normal everyday diet. Eating unusually large amounts of a suspect food can unbalance the test.

Test only a single suspect food at a time. And continue the test for a full 48 hours.

Keep a diary of foods eaten and of headache reactions. If the yellow cheese does not set off a headache, begin testing the next food on your list—say ice cream. Test it over the next 48 hours. Start with the food you suspect most and work down the list of suspect foods.

But what if the yellow cheese triggers a headache? In this case, you would stop eating it and return to your regular anti-migraine diet for the next four days. You would then commence to test the next suspect food on your list, ice cream. If after 48 hours, the ice cream did not precipitate a headache, you would return to testing the yellow cheese for a second time. You would test it for the next 48 hours. If the yellow cheese gave you another headache, this would confirm that yellow cheese is very likely a migraine trigger food for you. So you would eliminate it once more and return to testing, one by one, the remaining foods on your list.

Test not more than four foods in any one test period. After testing for a period of eight days, return to your regular anti-migraine diet for a four-day rest period. You may immediately add to your diet each and every food or beverage that has successfully passed your test. After resting for four days, you may then resume testing for another eight days.

If and when a headache occurs, which will often be late in the evening or early the next day, the probability is that it was set off by your most recent test food. If a certain food continually provokes a headache, this is almost certain proof that it is a migraine trigger.

After testing all the suspect foods on your list, you can begin to add back other foods by testing them, one at a time, for a 48-hour period. Eventually, you will have restored to your diet every food and beverage that is safe for you.

There's more good news. After eliminating a proven migraine trigger food for four months, you can reintroduce it into your diet on a rotational basis, that is, *once* every four days. Naturally, if it sets off a headache again, you would eliminate it permanently.

In some cases, chronic tension headaches have also been traced to food addiction. The possibility that headaches other than migraine may be related to food was emphasized by James M. Breneman M.D., when recently chairman of the Allergy Committee of the American College of Allergists. Dr. Breneman suggested that as many as 70 percent of all headaches might be traced to food sensitivities.

Once more, we emphasize that before making any dietary changes, you should consult your physician.

☐ Anti-Headache Technique #3-A: A Proven Remedy for Hypoglycemia Headache

Hypoglycemia, or low blood sugar, is one of the most common and dependable migraine triggers. It can also set off a less severe ''hunger'' headache in non-migraineurs.

Hypoglycemia can be caused in one of three ways: by skipping meals, especially breakfast; by dieting; and by eating meals high in refined carbohydrates (white flour, sugar and other sweeteners) along with fats and caffeine.

Hypoglycemia headaches frequently appear after sleeping late on weekend mornings and so failing to eat breakfast at the usual time. Skipping meals, or eating junk food on the run, are also common causes. Any foods high in white flour and sugar, or other sweeteners, when washed down with coffee or cola drinks, send blood sugar levels skyrocketing. We feel wonderfully alert and filled with energy.

But not for long!

The body consumes refined foods so swiftly that only an hour or so later, the blood sugar level plummets and we suddenly feel drained and depleted of energy. The low blood sugar causes our muscles to tense and this, in turn, sets off a reactive dilation in blood vessels in the head. Long before our next meal is due, we have a full-blown headache.

Fortunately, in most non-migraineurs, a hunger headache can be ended in a few minutes by drinking a large glass of orange or grapefruit juice. But fruit juice doesn't help once a migraine is triggered.

Luckily, hypoglycemia can be prevented altogether by adopting a simple three-step nutritional program. And whether your headaches are migraine or simple "hunger" headaches, both will vanish along with the hypoglycemia.

Here are the rules.

• Step 1. Get up at the same time every day and eat a full-sized breakfast. If you must sleep late on weekends, wake up at your usual breakfast hour, eat a snack, and return to sleep.

• Step 2. Eat all meals evenly spaced out and at usual meal hours. Avoid skipping any meals.

• Step 3. Eat a diet high in complex carbohydrates (meaning high in fiber) and low in fat. Stop all refined carbohydrates and drastically cut down on oils and fats. Instead, switch to fresh fruits and vegetables plus whole grains, seeds, and legumes. You may also have a small, once-daily serving of deep sea fish, or of chicken or turkey without the skin. Non-fat, plain yogurt or very low-fat cottage cheese are other good sources of whole protein.

Breakfast is the best time to eat fish, poultry or low-fat dairy products since animal protein is slow to digest and it helps stabilize blood sugar levels through much of the day. Fats of all kinds should be minimized as lipids can interfere with insulin metabolism, a condition that often leads to low blood sugar.

By contrast, a diet high in fiber stabilizes blood sugar levels and helps the body's insulin to function normally.

Three small surveys of hypoglycemic migraineurs made in Britain each showed that changing to a high-fiber, low-fat diet reduced incidence of migraine attacks by approximately 75 percent, and also diminished headache intensity.

☐ Anti-Headache Technique #4: Vitamin Strategy for Headache Relief

Taken together, vitamin C and a vitamin B-complex supplement are believed to work synergistically to achieve a level of muscle relaxation that has helped some women reduce the frequency and intensity of classic migraine attacks.

Several clinical ecologists have reported finding consistently low levels of B vitamins in chronic migraine sufferers, especially women. Although low levels of vitamins B_1, B_2 and B_5 can each contribute to headache risk, the key nutrient appears to be vitamin B_3, or niacin.

Niacin comes in two forms, niacin, also called nicotinic

acid, and niacinamide. The principal difference is that niacin causes a skin flush about 15 minutes after taking while niacinamide usually does not. Both types are freely available in health food stores in 50-milligram tablets. For headache therapy, niacinamide is usually recommended.

Although no studies have confirmed niacinamide's effectiveness, the literature contains numerous anecdotal reports in which niacinamide has been used successfully, both for long-term migraine prevention, and to abort a classic migraine attack. According to these reports, vitamin therapy seems to be most effective when used by female migraineurs.

For prevention, you can take 500 mg of vitamin C daily, together with the manufacturer's recommended dosage of a B-complex supplement that contains all the principal B vitamins, including niacin or niacinamide.

Even better results have been obtained by adding two heaping tablespoons of brewer's yeast to your breakfast cereal each morning; or by stirring it into a glass of orange juice. If, in addition, you eat plenty of other whole grain foods plus fresh fruits and vegetables each day, you should not need to take supplements of either vitamin C or the B vitamins. Brewer's yeast is an inexpensive nutrient available in every health food store. It is a rich source of B vitamins, including niacin. Naturally, if yeast is a migraine trigger for you, you will prefer to take supplements rather than brewer's yeast.

Whether you take brewer's yeast or a B-complex supplement daily it will be at least 15 days before the average migraineur begins replenishing her depleted store of B vitamins. So take it for several weeks before anticipating results.

In addition to using vitamins B and C prophylactically, some women have claimed that by taking a 50 mg tablet of niacinamide at the first hint of an approaching aura, they have aborted a classic migraine headache. We have also seen several reports in which women were able to abort classic migraine attacks by taking a regular vitamin B-complex supplement at the first sign of aura symptoms.

Niacinamide appears to work by dilating capillaries in the skin about 15 minutes after taking. This dilation, it has been suggested, could break up a migraine sequence in Stage 2.

Many approved stress formulas include 100 mg of daily niacinamide. At the daily amounts mentioned here, 500 mg for vitamin C and 50 mg for niacinamide, both vitamins are considered entirely safe. However, it is generally considered that no one should take more than 100 mg of niacinamide per day without a doctor's supervision.

If you have any kind of health problem, or are taking any kind of medication, you should see your doctor before taking vitamins or changing your diet. Naturally, should any adverse side effects appear, such as itchy skin, nausea or red patches in the skin, you should immediately discontinue taking niacinamide or other vitamins.

Since B vitamins work more effectively when the entire complex is present, a single B-complex supplement is preferable to taking separate amounts of each B vitamin.

Obviously, vitamin therapy isn't going to stop migraine in everyone. But expensive and toxic drugs are not always successful either. Taking vitamins prophylactically, especially in the form of food, is a low-cost natural therapy available to everyone without risk or inconvenience.

☐ Anti-Headache Technique #4-A: A Natural Muscle Relaxant That May Prevent Migraine

After reading the results of two university studies made during the mid-1980s, thousands of women migraine sufferers have diminished their migraine symptoms by taking daily magnesium supplements.

In the first study, at East Tennessee State University, 500 selected women with migraine were each asked to take 100 or 200 mg of magnesium in supplement form daily. For some, relief came within hours. Most felt much better in just a few days. Some women, who had had splitting headaches for two straight weeks, quickly became symptom-free. Overall, seven out of ten women had no migraines for as long as they continued taking the magnesium.

In a similar study reported from Case Western Reserve, headaches stopped in 80 percent of sufferers after they had taken 200 mg of supplemental magnesium for two or three weeks. In another case, a Chicago woman who had suffered migraine attacks several times weekly for over ten years, had had to take increasing amounts of drugs to control her pain. Agony and depression were wrecking her life. Yet after taking 200 mg of supplemental magnesium daily for four weeks, her headaches had almost completely disappeared.

It has been suggested that, through causing the smooth muscles surrounding each artery in the body to relax and dilate, magnesium effectively blocks Stage 2 in the migraine sequence.

Other studies have shown that four out of every five Americans are deficient in magnesium reserves, especially those who drink soda or alcoholic beverages. Many drugs also bind with magnesium and prevent its absorption.

Magnesium supplements in 200 mg tablets are readily available in any health food store. An intake of 200 mg a day is considered riskless by most nutritionists. However, if you have any kidney or other health problems, or are under medical treatment or taking medication, you should consult your physician before taking supplemental magnesium.

Alternatively, you can increase your dietary uptake of magnesium by eating more magnesium-rich foods such as avocados, soybeans, black-eyed peas, almonds, cashews, Brazil nuts and other types of beans and peas.

☐ Anti-Headache Technique #5: Headache Freedom Through Tryptophan Loading

A theory becoming increasingly popular in pain clinics is that foods containing tryptophan may offer a safe and effective nutritional approach to headache relief.

The rationale is that tryptophan, an essential amino acid, is a precursor of serotonin, a neurotransmitter essential to pain control.

Serotonin plays a dual role in the headache process:

• In response to emotional stress, blood platelets coagulate and release serotonin into the bloodstream. This serotonin constricts blood vessels and can readily precipitate Stage 2 in the migraine process.

• Serotonin is also released in the brain where it acts as an effective sedative, painkiller and antidepressant. In tandem with norepinephrine, serotonin limits passage of pain impulses through the brain's "pain gate."

By enhancing enkephalin and endorphin activity, brain serotonin also raises the pain threshold and blocks pain impulses. Serotonin is also a natural tranquilizer that encourages sleep and it helps to relieve mild depression and anxiety.

Availability of serotonin in the brain is largely dependent on dietary sources of tryptophan. In many people, tryptophan has difficulty penetrating the blood-brain barrier, a protective biochemical shield. Tryptophan is prevented from reaching the brain by a flood of competing amino acids, most of which are released from foods of animal origin. People with the lowest levels of brain serotonin are likely to be heavy eaters of meat, poultry, eggs, cheese and other whole milk dairy products.

This may sound contradictory, since these same foods are also rich sources of tryptophan. The problem is that each also contains even higher amounts of other amino acids, all of which compete with tryptophan for transportation through the blood-brain barrier. Additionally, many animal foods contain large amounts of saturated fats, which stimulate release of a prostaglandin that thickens blood and, indirectly, may assist platelets to clot and release serotonin.

Animal experiments by Drs. Wurtman and Fernstrom of M.I.T. a few years ago revealed that a diet high in complex carbohydrates, and low in fats and animal protein, is best for helping tryptophan to reach the brain.

However, except for beans, tryptophan exists only in foods of animal origin. The safest and best of these tryptophan sources is plain, nonfat yogurt, skimmed buttermilk, very low-fat cottage cheese, and nonfat or skim milk. Worthwhile amounts of tryptophan also exist in oily fish such as mackerel, sardines, salmon, haddock, cod and canned tuna. Oily fish of this type also contain EPA (eicosapentaenoic acid) which, unlike saturated fat, actually thins blood and inhibits platelets from clumping and releasing serotonin.

Undoubtedly, the foods just mentioned are the safest sources of dietary tryptophan. Tryptophan also exists in whole-milk-dairy foods, poultry, meat and in non-oily fish.

The most effective way to boost brain tryptophan intake is to eat one or more helpings of the recommended tryptophan-rich foods at dinner. It is not necessary or desirable to eat larger-than-normal helpings.

How Natural Foods Provide Headache Relief

The trick now is to liberate the tryptophan from the protein in these foods and make it accessible to the brain.

You do that by eating a late-night snack consisting solely of complex carbohydrates. Although the actual mechanism by which a vegetarian snack provides tryptophan with priority transportation to the brain remains a mystery, its effectiveness has been amply demonstrated by numerous insomnia researchers.

Serotonin also promotes sleep. And sleep clinics use this same nutritional technique to get tryptophan through the blood-brain barrier of their insomnia patients late in the day.

Either sweet or starchy complex carbohydrates will release tryptophan and speed it to the brain. Among sweet carbohydrates are apples, bananas, dates, pears, raisins or melons. Starchy carbohydrates that work well include beans, corn, oatmeal, parsnips, peas, potatoes, brown rice, sweet potatoes, whole grains (including bread) and winter squash.

For example, dinner might include baked cod with steamed potatoes, corn and brown rice together with a slice of whole grain bread spread with soft avocado and eaten with a small cup of plain nonfat yogurt. For a late night-snack, you might try a sandwich of whole-grain bread spread with avocado, using a banana as filler. The bread should be 100 percent whole-grain and free of oils, fats or sweeteners. Most health food stores carry such breads. Or you could use pita bread made exclusively of whole-grain flour. (Be warned that most "whole-grain" breads on supermarket shelves are made "with" not "exclusively of" whole grains, and the majority are made with fats, oils or sweeteners.)

A Nutrient That May Block Headaches in Stage Four

While it is obviously wisest to obtain as much tryptophan as possible from the diet, some nutritionists have recommended taking an additional one gram daily in the form of L-tryptophan supplements. Until late 1989, these were available over the counter in most healthfood stores. However, at that time they were linked to a rare blood disorder called eosinophilia. Most L-tryptophan supplements were immediately recalled, and all stocks have since been removed from store shelves. When and if the FDA concludes that they are not the cause of eosinophilia, and are once more considered safe, they may again become available.

Should this occur, you will want to know that L-tryptophan supplements are usually available in 250 or 500 mg tablets. They metabolize rapidly in the bloodstream and can induce drowsiness within 30 minutes. Drowsiness, incidentally, is a good sign that tryptophan has reached the brain and has broken down into serotonin. For this reason, tryptophan nutrition is best carried out just prior to bedtime.

Most nutritionists suggest that, without medical supervision, tryptophan supplements should be limited to a maximum of one gram per day. (However, manufacturer's labels have suggested that up to two grams may be taken.) Naturally, if any adverse side effects occur, dosage should be terminated immediately. In practice, adverse side effects are extremely unlikely but very large doses could possibly cause bladder problems. As pain tolerance increases, most nutritionists recommend reducing intake of supplements and relying, if possible, on dietary sources alone.

Prolonged intake of L-tryptophan may lead to depletion of vitamin B_6. Too, a sufficiency of vitamin B_3 is necessary to maintain tryptophan levels in the brain.

For optimum results, when and if L-tryptophan supplements again become available, it would seem best to combine tryptophan nutrition with daily supplements of vitamins C and the B complex as described earlier in this chapter.

Since it blocks headache pain in Stage 4, tryptophan therapy works equally well for all types of headaches. Best results have been reported with tension and migraine headaches.

☐ Anti-Headache Technique #5-A: How to Avoid Ice Cream Headache

If eating ice cream, or other very cold foods, gives you a headache, it's due to their contact with nerves in the roof of your mouth and in the throat areas.

Here's how to avoid it. Eat the ice cream slowly and in small amounts so that it melts easily in the mouth and does not impact the roof of the mouth or throat with large, icy chunks. It's also a good idea to wait a few minutes and allow the ice cream to warm up to a creamy consistency before eating. Many people also swear it tastes better when warmed a few degrees.

However, some migraineurs have told us that, by holding ice cream in the mouth, they are able to abort a migraine. Apparently, what works for Peter does not always work for Paul.

After reading this far, you have probably noticed an outstanding fact about headache nutrition. It is that a vegetarian, or near-vegetarian, diet almost invariably leads to a steady reduction in headache pain. By practicing the nutritional therapies in this chapter, you may well find that relief from headache lies right in your own kitchen.

6 The Herbal Approach

For years, computer programmer Betty Schreiner of San Antonio, Texas suffered from chronic migraine headaches that kept her indoors for days at a time.

One day at a party, she met a lady from Germany whose hobby was herbal medicine. When Betty told the herbalist about her endless migraines, the German lady advised Betty to take a capsule of feverfew each day as a prophylactic measure. Feverfew, the herbalist explained, is a rather bitter-tasting herb that is conveniently available in taste-free capsule form in health food stores.

The very next day, Betty bought a supply of feverfew capsules and began taking them prophylactically.

"Just as the herbalist lady predicted, my headaches began to disappear," Betty told us later. "After taking a daily capsule for three weeks, my headaches had diminished to almost nothing. I used to just want to curl up and die. But feverfew has become my assurance of headache relief."

☐ Anti-Headache Technique #6: Herbal Relief for Migraine Pain

Feverfew is the only herb to have been scientifically validated as an effective headache remedy. Two studies conducted at the City of London Migraine Clinic in England have suggested that feverfew is effective in reducing severity and frequency of migraine.

In the first study, researchers analyzed questionnaires from 300 migraine sufferers who had been taking feverfew daily for an average period of two and a half years. Since taking feverfew, 30 percent reported complete cessation of all headaches, 70 percent reported that attacks were less frequent and less painful, and 40 percent reported less muscular pain and better sleep. Most respondents were consuming feverfew in its natural leaf form, eating three small leaves or one large leaf daily.

In the second study, 17 people were selected from 270 chronic migraine sufferers, each of whom had been taking feverfew daily in the form of fresh leaves for at least three months.

Eight of the selected patients continued to take freeze-dried feverfew in capsule form while the remaining 9 patients received a placebo. Six months later, patients receiving the placebo were suffering an average of 3.4 migraines per month, and those receiving feverfew only 1.5 per month.

After the study, all 17 patients were given placebos and within a few weeks, all were experiencing an average 3.43 headaches per month. Still later, all returned to taking feverfew and their headache average dropped back to only 1.5 per month.

In reporting the study in the *British Medical Journal* (August 31, 1985), the authors concluded that feverfew taken prophylactically can undoubtedly prevent migraine attack. But, they added, it is not known with certainty that feverfew is safe for long-term use. Nor does feverfew help everyone.

How a Simple Herb Can Stop the Migraine Process

Still another British study made at University Hospital, Nottingham, identified the active ingredients in feverfew as parthenolide and sesquiterpene lactone. These agents apparently block the headache process in Stage 2. First, they inhibit platelet coagulation, which stops secretion of serotonin. This serotonin would otherwise lock into receptors in smooth muscle cells surrounding arteries in the head and cause them to constrict. To make doubly sure this does not happen, the feverfew ingredients also lock on to these receptors, thus preventing access of serotonin. For good measure, the agents also inhibit release of prostaglandin, another essential step in the headache sequence.

Since results of these studies were released, feverfew has become popular with thousands of British migraineurs who normally would have taken aspirin but who were unable to tolerate the gastrointestinal side effects.

A common plant of the chrysanthemum family, feverfew has been used to treat migraine since medieval times. It may also have other benefits. Sixty percent of British migraineurs taking feverfew reported that they felt much more relaxed, experienced less tension, and slept better. Meanwhile, migraineurs who also had rheumatoid arthritis reported diminished arthritic pain.

The Number One Herb For Headache Relief

Feverfew is sold throughout Europe in drug and health food stores in both tablet and capsule forms, and is also becoming available in U.S. health food stores. Because the tablets are bitter and have a camphorlike taste, capsules are the preferred way to take feverfew.

In the London trials, dosage was two 50 mg capsules per day. But many Britons reported that three capsules gave better results. Feverfew capsules in U.S. stores typically contain as much as 340 mg and a single capsule per day is usually recommended on the label.

To be sure that you are taking authentic feverfew, check that the botanical name is *Chrysanthemum parthenium*. Leaves in capsules should be freeze-dried rather than air- or sun-dried.

Fresh feverfew leaves may also be used if available. Like the tablets, they are bitter-tasting and have a camphorlike smell. To mask the disagreeable taste, the yellow-green leaves are usually eaten in a sandwich spread with butter and honey. You can use one large leaf, two medium-sized leaves or three to four small leaves. This constitutes the dosage for one day.

Feverfew leaves are also dried and powdered and sold as a tea. Herbalists recommend steeping half a teaspoon to a teaspoon of this tea in a cup of boiling water and drinking two to three cups daily.

Although side effects with capsules are minor, approximately 18 percent of Britons who took feverfew in leaf form reported allergic reactions in mouth and tongue. In some cases, direct contact with feverfew leaves caused mouth ulcers to appear. They cleared up quickly when feverfew was stopped. Feverfew can also reduce blood pressure, stimulate appetite and cause diarrhea. The City of London Migraine Clinic has advised against its use by pregnant women, though no evidence of any risk has been found.

After taking feverfew over a long period, withdrawal symptoms such as nervousness, insomnia and joint stiffness may appear. Most pharmacists equate feverfew's toxicity to that of coffee. However, the long-term toxicity of fever-few remains unknown.

Herbals For Headaches

While most doctors scorn herbal remedies, they are, according to the World Health Organization, still used as primary treatment for half the world's population. Considering the mediocre record of pharmaceutical drugs, it seems that herbal remedies are often as effective and in some cases more so. Indeed, some contemporary drugs, such as digitalis, are still derived from herbs.

But nowadays, pharmaceutical companies prefer to use chemical analogs so that they can manipulate active ingredients to minimize side effects, as well as to secure patent rights and to lengthen shelf life. Thus mainstream medicine continues to ignore herbs. The FDA regards them as food. And the majority remain unregulated and freely available.

Although herbs are natural, organic alternatives to drugs—with side effects, if any, that are mild by comparison—care is required for self-medication. For example, if one cup of a herb tea per day is beneficial, it doesn't follow that three cups is better. Nor should herbs ever be smoked. As previously stated, the long-term effects of taking most herbs has not been studied.

Nowadays, most larger health food stores have a herbal section with a wide array of herbs and herb teas, both in bulk and packaged. But it is often hard to find herbs in smaller towns.

Herbs for headache relief usually work prophylactically and you may have to take the remedy for several weeks before optimal results appear. Nowadays, too, most herbalists prefer to prescribe a blend of several herbs in order to broaden the treatment. Most herbal remedies for migraine use feverfew as the core but add other herbs like sage or skullcap which are believed to be powerful artery constrictors.

More Healing Herbs to Beat Headache Pain

Other herbs frequently prescribed to augment feverfew are camomile, a nervous system relaxant; ginseng, a nullifier of stress symptoms; hawthorn leaf, which may soothe cerebral arteries; rosemary and lemon balm, believed to prevent nausea; wild yam, said to help menstrual migraines; dandelion root, believed to minimize allergic reactions; and willow bark, a recognized painkiller containing chemicals similar to aspirin. Peppermint, cayenne, fennel, hops, catnip and echinacea are also used as headache remedies.

The most popular way to take herbs is in the form of a tea. Make a fairly strong brew, equivalent to infusing one teabag of black tea in a cup of boiling water. Since some medicinal herbs have a bitter taste, you may add lemon, honey or a pleasant-tasting herb tea to improve the taste.

Packaged herbal mixes are also often available. Since herbs are classed as foods, they cannot bear labels describing them as therapeutic. Yet there is one exception. Herbal remedies distributed by FDA-licensed drug companies are free of this restriction. Currently, packaged herbals are distributed by several FDA-licensed drug companies, including Nature's Way, McZand and Traditional Herbs. Their products use FDA-approved ingredients and the labels prescribe an FDA-approved safe dose.

Among packaged herbals helpful for headaches are antistress herbal formulas which combine herbs like valerian, skullcap and passion flower with minerals such as magnesium and calcium, and also with amino acids. Designed to relax the nervous system and muscles, these mixes can be useful as prophylactics for chronic tension and migraine headaches.

Among other promising herbal remedies is a tea imported from China consisting of magnolia and petafolia blossom teas. According to studies made in the People's Republic of China, this tea provides dramatic relief for chronic tension headaches.

☐ Anti-Headache Technique #6-A: Help from Homeopathy

Herbs and other naturally occurring substances are also used in treating headaches with homeopathic medicines. As more and more Americans lose confidence in conventional medical care, they are assuming responsibility for their own health and are turning to new and alternative healing options. The most popular alternative to drug therapy is homeopathic medicine.

Homeopathy uses a number of natural medicines. When given in large doses, these medicines tend to produce side effects. The side effects, or symptoms, of all homeopathic medicines have been carefully observed and catalogued over many years. The principle behind homeopathy is to treat a patient's symptoms with a homeopathic medicine that produces the same symptoms. The rationale is that when given in very small doses, a well-chosen medication can cure illnesses that have similar symptoms.

Homeopathic medicines are best prescribed by a homeopathic physician. In determining a patient's symptom profile, a homeopathic physician will consider not only physical but psychological and even spiritual symptoms. Thus homeopathy is clearly holistic. Symptoms are regarded as evidence of the body-mind's attempts to heal itself. The right homeopathic medicine will stimulate those symptoms and speed the healing process.

Natural Medicines May Be Superior

Before dismissing homeopathy as unscientific, we should not forget that the adverse side effects of many pharmaceuticals include symptoms of the very disease that the drugs are prescribed to cure. Certain drugs prescribed for headaches can cause more headaches in some people. Likewise, some drugs and treatments prescribed to cure cancer may actually cause more cancer than they cure.

Unlike modern-day herbalists who tend to prescribe a mix of herbs, homeopathic physicians prescribe a single remedy. That remedy is then given in frugal amounts to match the totality of Whole Person symptoms. For successful homeopathic diagnosis and treatment, you should consult a licensed homeopathic physician. Nonetheless, due to opposition from mainstream medicine, most Americans have been deprived of access to a licensed homeopathic physician. As a result, tens of thousands of Americans, disillusioned with allopathy, are being forced to practice do-it-yourself homeopathy. Nowadays, many health food stores, as well as some drug stores, carry a full range of homeopathic OTC remedies.

To make prescribing easier, a variety of homeopathic health care kits is appearing together with packaged OTC homeopathic medicines. Some of these packaged medicines are combinations of various homeopathic substances. This commercial shotgun approach directly contradicts one of homeopathy's cardinal principles, which is to select a single remedy.

Another important homeopathic principle is that the more times a medicine is diluted, the more potent it becomes. While this also may sound illogical, let's not forget that fewer than 15 percent of all medical treatments have been scientifically validated by controlled studies. And Paul Pearsall, Ph.D. reminds us in his book *Superimmunity*

(Ballantine, 1987) that out of every ten people who see a medical doctor: eight neither get better nor worse as a result of medical intervention; one gets worse—often with the help of a new disease induced by a drug prescribed by the doctor; and only one out of ten (ten percent) actually benefits from medical treatment.

Using Non-Pharmaceutical Medicines

With help from books and from health food store personnel, thousands of Americans are successfully treating themselves with homeopathic medicines and far more than ten percent are actually receiving benefit. One reason is that, used in correct amounts, homeopathic remedies are too weak to cause any harm.

In making your personal symptom profile, use only the strongest and clearest headache symptoms. You must then find a medicine with a match for your symptoms

A homeopathic physician will typically prescribe a dose to be taken about once every two hours. If improvement appears, you stop taking the medicine and do not resume again unless improvement ceases or symptoms become worse. In either case, if there is no improvement after two to three doses, most homeopathic physicians would probably change to another medicine which matches your symptoms as closely as possible.

Among homeopathic medicines most widely prescribed for headache by homeopathic physicians are these (with symptoms as described in standard homeopathic literature):

- *Belladonna* causes headache symptoms that closely resemble those of migraine or cluster headaches, namely a pounding pain that feels better when sitting and worsens on exertion and that may include a hot and flushed face.

- *Bryonia* causes headaches with symptoms that resemble a tension headache. A Bryonia headache is worsened by moving about and often extends from the forehead up and over the scalp and down to the neck. A Bryonia headache often leads to irritability and a preference for being alone.

• *Gelsemium* creates a headache similar to that of classic migraine. It extends from the back of the head over the scalp and down to the forehead. A Gelsemium headache is often worsened by noise, light or motion. The person's eyes droop, and he or she prefers to rest and be alone.

• *Iris* creates a headache very similar to that of periodic classic migraine, complete with visual disturbances, and with pain experienced on one side of the head only. Nausea and vomiting are also common.

• *Nux Vomica* causes a headache similar to that produced by a hangover or by caffeine withdrawal or drugs. The headaches are worst on awakening and gradually improve through the day. Other symptoms include irascibility and irritation. Shaking the head worsens a Nux Vomica headache.

• *Pulsatilla* creates a vascular type of headache similar to that produced by food allergies or by menstrual migraines. It is a pulsating pain, located either in the forehead or in one temple or eye, and it can lead to nausea and vomiting.

• *Spigelia* creates a headache similar to that of a cluster with severe throbbing pain around one eye and deep into the socket. The pain is often on the left side of the head, it worsens with motion, and the head and neck often become stiff. A Spigelia headache often worsens in warm weather and improves in cold weather.

• *Sanguinaria* creates a migraine-style headache that begins at the back of the neck and reaches up over the scalp to the right eye and temple. The stabbing pain is as intense as in a cluster headache and it frequently provokes nausea and vomiting. Sanguinaria is often prescribed for vascular headaches that appear regularly at periodic intervals, such as once a week.

We recommend that you consult an experienced herbalist, or a licensed naturopath or homeopathic physician, before trying to treat yourself. But because herbs and homeopathic medicines are seldom dangerous in moderate amounts, risk of harm is slight.

The important thing is to have already read Chapter 2 and to ensure that your headache really is benign before you try any alternative healing method. Otherwise, herbs or homeopathy could delay you from receiving essential emergency medical treatment.

7 The Physical Approach

Arlene W., a Denver housewife, had suffered for years from the unremitting pain of agonizing tension headaches. That is, until she accompanied her husband on a business trip to Taiwan. On her first day in Taipei, the capital, she was confined to bed with a disabling headache. The hotel doctor turned out to be an older Chinese who spoke English fluently.

"I can give you a modern analgesic that will merely relieve pain," he said. "Or I can show you an ancient Chinese technique through which you can rid yourself of headaches for the rest of your life."

Despite her persistent pain, Arlene opted for the Li-Shou technique.

☐ Anti-Headache Technique #7: The Li-Shou Method

All she had to do, Arlene found, was to stand up with feet about twenty inches apart and rub her hands together until the palms were warm. Then, using her warm palms, she was to lightly stroke her face from brow to chin 30 times in the same direction.

Next, still standing, she was to partially close her eyes, look down at her feet, and continue to hold this stance throughout the exercise. Following this, she was to extend her arms out in front at waist level with fingers touching. Then she was instructed to swing her arms back behind her until her fingers touched, and then to swing her arms out in front again. She was to do 100 of these arm swings. Throughout, she must keep her awareness focused on her toes and not allow her thoughts to wander.

Before the count of 100, Arlene realized that the awful pain in her head had completely disappeared. Since then, for more than a year, she has practiced Li-shou every morning before breakfast—and she has not had a single headache.

Li-Shou, which means "hand swinging" in Chinese, is highly effective because swinging the arms shunts blood away from dilated arteries in the head and into the arms. Simultaneously, the exercise releases endorphins in the brain that also help to relieve pain.

As additional blood is drawn from the head into the hands and arms, the arteries dilate and the hands and arms become warmer. This is the same effect as that achieved through biofeedback. By keeping the awareness on the toes, this condition is then transferred to the feet, which also become warmer.

After practicing Li-Shou for two or three weeks, arteries in both hands and feet remain dilated throughout the day. By redirecting the blood flow away from the head, the Li-Shou method makes further headaches almost impossible.

Li-Shou works well for both tension and migraine headaches, both as a prophylactic and to abort a headache which has already occurred. As a prophylactic, it should be practiced once a day. When stroking the face, avoid touching the eyes. Simply stroke the flat of the face lightly with your palms. Don't rub or press hard on the face. Naturally, if you have any ill effects from the exercise, you should stop at once.

Physical Therapy Can Conquer Most Headaches

As explained in Chapter 1, emotional stress is the underlying cause of most headaches. In a headache-prone person, this psychological stress is swiftly transformed into physical stress mechanisms that affect posture and create tension or spasm in muscles, particularly in those enclosing blood vessels, and in the neck and shoulders. These distortions of body mechanics then set off a muscle-contraction headache, or they may act as a trigger for migraine.

Relief is often as easy as brisk, rhythmic exercise, deep breathing, stretching, brushing or massaging, and using acupressure or at-home heat and cold treatment. Although these physical therapies are completely harmless for most healthy people, you are advised to consult your doctor before beginning any of the physical therapies described in this chapter.

☐ Anti-Headache Technique #7-A: A Simple Stretching Technique That Relieves Tension Headache

Developed in the early 1980s by neurologists at Loma Linda University in California, this technique has successfully ended chronic tension headache in 90 percent of sufferers.

The tension technique is simplicity itself. You merely sit upright in a chair and:

1. Turn your head to the left as though looking back over the left shoulder.

2. Place your left index finger on the right cheek with palm and thumb under chin. Very gently, push the head to the left.

3. Simultaneously, place the right hand on top of the head with the middle finger touching the top of the left ear.

4. Very gently, exert pressure with your right hand to pull the head down towards the chest. Just before you feel any discomfort, stop at that point and hold for ten seconds. Then release.

5. Repeat on the right side.

6. Repeat twice more on each side for a total of six neck stretches, three on each side.

Be very gentle. *Do not push or pull hard or force anything.* Simply apply very gentle, steady pressure and do not go beyond the point where discomfort begins. Should you experience any pain or discomfort, or feel dizzy, discontinue the technique.

Neck stretching was developed after neurologists discovered that taut neck muscles are the mechanical cause of most tension headaches. As you exert gentle pressure with your hands, you should feel the taut muscle and fibrous tissue in your neck being stretched and released.

To relieve chronic tension headache, one series of six neck stretches as just described should be done once every two hours during the day. After the headache is relieved, neck stretching can be continued twice a day as a prophylactic measure. The complete technique takes only two minutes to accomplish.

Headache clinics report that most people with chronic tension headaches usually feel much better after only a single week of neck stretching. Within six weeks, approximately half of all sufferers have reported complete freedom from chronic tension headaches. And within three months, all but the most stubborn cases have usually disappeared.

Neck stretching can also provide quick relief from acute tension headache—the occasional tension headaches experienced by millions daily. It has also helped victims of common migraine.

Alternatively, any combination of neck rolls, or moving of the head from side to side, or up and down, or turning from left to right and vice versa, plus shoulder shrugs and shoulder rotations, can benefit tension headaches. However, people with arthritis or stiff necks may prefer to use massage, brushing, or heat or cold treatment.

☐ Anti-Headache Technique #8: Walk Your Headache Away

Whether to abort an existing headache or to prevent future headaches, brisk rhythmic exercise is one of the most successful natural headache therapies. It is equally effective for tension, migraine or cluster headache and it also defuses stress, anxiety and depression. (To abort a cluster see Technique #8-A.)

At least ten studies have demonstrated that half an hour of brisk daily exercise such as walking stimulates the anterior-pituitary gland to secrete beta-endorphin, one of the natural opiates discussed in Chapter 3 that prevents headache pain from being experienced. The studies also found that exercise raises self-esteem, lessens anxiety, relieves depression, improves oxygen uptake and cerebral functioning, and creates an upbeat mood that lasts for 24 hours.

Several of the studies showed that a brisk half-hour walk also suppresses a number of migraine trigger mechanisms. For example, a small study of nine sedentary migraineurs at the University of Wisconsin found that after 15 weeks of walking and running, the group's frequency of headaches had fallen by 50 percent. And if a migraine did occur, its severity was greatly diminished.

Some researchers have concluded that a migraine headache can never reach full intensity in a person who exercises daily. Furthermore, exercise can be used to abort a migraine provided it is begun at the first hint of an approaching headache. Although exercise is a powerful vasodilator, it apparently prevents blood vessels from reaching the excessive stage of dilation which causes migraine and tension headache pain.

To abort either a migraine or tension headache, resist any temptation to lie down. Instead, begin to walk briskly out of doors. If this is not possible, pedal a stationary bicycle (near an open window in mild weather), or swim, or walk briskly up and down stairs. Very often within 20 minutes the headache will have partially or fully disappeared.

Although brisk walking is probably best, any rhythmic exercise will bring additional endorphins flooding into the brain to clear your head. For some people, brisk walking is the only therapy that will completely eliminate a stubborn headache.

You may feel a little groggy after walking off a severe migraine attack. But as a rule, 20 minutes of brisk walking is enough to make the headache itself disappear completely.

To increase the effectiveness of walking therapy, swing the arms vigorously up to shoulder height. This gives a gentle massage to stiff neck and shoulder muscles and relaxes the entire neck area as you walk.

Some headaches are so incapacitating that exercising would be impossible. Even with one of these headsplitters, you will recover faster if you can go outdoors and walk as soon as the pain begins to subside.

A brisk daily walk of half an hour or longer is an excellent prophylactic for all headache types—muscle-contraction, migraine or cluster.

The exercise you choose must be brisk and it must provide an unbroken pattern of rhythmic movement. Walking is ideal because it needs no equipment, is unlikely to cause injury, and requires no prior warm-up or stretching. By contrast, stop-and-go exercises like baseball, doubles tennis, bowling or golf create so little extra oxygen uptake that they cannot be seriously considered for either short- or long-term exercise therapy.

Obviously, if you are not sufficiently fit or in shape to be able to walk briskly for at least half an hour, you should not suddenly begin to walk as a headache therapy. If you are over 35, overweight, smoke or drink alcohol, are unfit or sedentary, or have any disorder or dysfunction that may be worsened by exercise, you should see your doctor before undertaking any form of exercise therapy.

On the other hand, if you enjoy brisk walking or other forms of aerobic exercise, you don't have to stop after half an hour. Long walks of one to two hours or more can be even more beneficial.

☐ Anti-Headache Technique #8-A: Giving the One-Two Punch to Cluster Headache

Cluster headaches occur when arteries in the head overdilate in response to a lack of oxygen in the bloodstream. When pure oxygen is inhaled, the arteries return to normal size in just a few minutes and the headache is aborted.

Since vigorous exercise dramatically boosts oxygen uptake, it follows that any type of active, rhythmic exercise should stop a cluster as effectively as oxygen. And, indeed, this is perfectly correct. Any fairly vigorous exercise, such as jogging, usually stops a cluster headache within a few minutes.

The snag is that many cluster victims tend to be sedentary males who are often heavy smokers and whose breathing ability is already impaired. Instead of exercising, these cluster victims are advised to sit down and do a deep-breathing technique.

Only if you are physically fit and accustomed to vigorous exercise should you attempt to abort a cluster by active exercise. In any event, you should have your doctor's permission before attempting either form of behavioral therapy described below.

• *Deep Breathing Technique.* At the first hint of an impending cluster headache, sit in a chair with your spine straight, and begin a series of long, deep breaths. Breathe steadily and do not hold the breath at any point. Fill the bottom of the lungs first and then fill the top of the lungs by expanding the chest. When you exhale, squeeze the abdominal muscle to expel more air from the bottom of the lungs.

If you begin to feel dizzy, slow the rate of breathing slightly. If dizziness persists, or if you have any other adverse effects, discontinue the technique.

As the long, deep breaths bring a sufficiency of oxygen to the arteries in your head, the blood vessels will return to normal size and the headache will generally disappear. This usually takes only a few minutes.

Although this technique is primarily for those unable to exercise, it can also be used by all cluster victims. However, if the headache intensifies, those able to exercise should begin to do so.

• *Exercising Technique.* Any kind of vigorous exercise that raises the pulse rate to 120 beats per minute for 5–10 minutes will usually stop a cluster dead in its tracks. Exercise can consist of running or jogging, running in place, riding a stationary bicycle, or running up and down stairs. Ordinary walking, which seldom raises the pulse rate above 100 beats per minute, is not usually vigorous enough. However, race walking (heel-and-toe walking) works well.

Since you won't want to stop exercising to take your pulse during a cluster attack, you should undertake a few trial sessions beforehand to determine how vigorously you need to exercise to raise your pulse rate to 120 beats per minute for 5–10 minutes.

Incidentally, no one over 60 should attempt this technique since a heartbeat of 120 may exceed the upper limit considered safe in aerobic training.

For either the breathing or exercise techniques to work, they must be commenced *immediately* a cluster strikes, preferably within a few seconds. When exercising, it's best to stay close to home or the workplace in case the headache intensifies. Naturally, you would stop exercising at once if any adverse effects are perceived.

Cluster victims should also note that a brisk daily walking program, when maintained as a long-term prophylactic measure, can improve oxygen uptake to the point where cluster headaches are very unlikely ever to occur again. For details, see Anti-Headache Technique #8.

☐ Anti-Headache Technique #9: Breathe Away Migraines

If begun at the first hint of an impending aura, bag breathing can squelch classic migraine attacks within 10 to 20 minutes. It has also proved quite effective against common migraine.

This simple technique is based on the principle that carbon dioxide is a blood vessel dilator with the ability to release constricted arteries in Stage 2 of the migraine sequence.

We can easily direct carbon dioxide into the lungs and the bloodstream by breathing into and out of a brown paper bag. The oxygen in the bag is quickly used up and carbon dioxide takes its place.

To accomplish this, you simply squeeze the mouth of a medium-sized brown paper bag into a reasonably round hole shape, place your mouth over it, and start to breathe into and out of the paper bag. Remove your mouth from the bag only when the air becomes too stale to continue breathing. Allow some fresh air to enter your lungs, then continue to breathe into the bag.

Breathe deeply and slowly into the bag. The average migraineur should experience relief within 10 to 20 minutes.

Bag breathing works by releasing the constricted arteries of Stage 2. However, actual headache pain is not felt until the arteries suddenly dilate and Stage 3 begins. To be effective, bag breathing must be practiced during Stage 2; once Stage 3 commences, it's too late. Bag breathing then may *intensify* rather than relieve the headache.

This can be tricky, because no pain is experienced during Stage 2. In classic migraine, aura effects occur for 20 or 30 minutes during Stage 2. *By commencing bag breathing at the first hint of an aura*, the majority of classic migraines can be aborted while still in Stage 2.

Many sufferers from common migraine also learn to recognize the advance warnings of an impending headache. These, too, are often experienced early in Stage 2. If you are very quick, and begin to bag breathe at the very first hint of a common migraine, there's a good chance you can abort this type of headache also. Once the constricted arteries are released back to their normal size, they will not overdilate and the migraine sequence is broken.

Once you feel actual headache pain, bag breathing must

be stopped immediately. Otherwise, it could intensify Stage 3 dilation. And *never* use a plastic bag. Stop immediately if you experience any pain or discomfort. We recommend that you consult your physician before trying bag breathing and that you have him show you exactly how it is done.

These caveats aside, bag breathing has recently become such a popular therapy with classic migraineurs in Britain that thousands now carry a brown paper bag with them wherever they go.

☐ Anti-Headache Technique #9-A: Rub Away Headache Pain

You can literally rub away many headache pains by using self-massage or, even better, by having someone else massage you. Massage works because it increases blood flow to the painful area. It also helps to normalize muscle tone and blood vessel diameter in the afflicted area. Here are several massage techniques known to be effective for relief from tension or migraine headaches.

• *Massaging the Thumbs*. Rub the top joint of one of your thumbs vigorously for exactly 1½ minutes. Then repeat with the other thumb. Continue to alternate back and forth for a total of ˜12 minutes. Frequently, this is enough to relieve all but the most stubborn tension or migraine headache. If your headache has partially diminished yet still lingers on, continue the massage for another three minutes. Should your thumbs become sore, coat both fingers and thumb with baby oil or hand lotion before rubbing.

Several prominent neurologists have suggested that neural stimulation from the thumbs overloads the brain's pain control gate, preventing headache pain from being perceived in the brain.

• *Massaging the Neck*. Sit at a table. Support your forehead with your right hand, elbow on table. Then massage the muscle at the back of the neck between thumb and forefingers of your left hand. Using a circular motion, squeeze and massage each muscle on each side of your neck. Work slowly up and down the neck. Apply the same treatment to your shoulder muscles. Finally, give the scalp a vigorous rub with your knuckles and then with your fingertips, using a circular motion. Change hands frequently to prevent fatigue.

Alternatively, or in addition, dig the fingers of both hands into the groove at the back of your neck and massage the neck muscles between fingers and thumbs. Work up and down the neck the length of the groove for about three minutes. This relaxes the muscles of the upper neck and relieves the tension that causes muscular-contraction headaches.

• *Press Your Headaches Away.* Headache pain in the temples can often be relieved by pressing the temples with the palms, or with any firm object such as a tightly-folded cold damp washcloth. So effective is this technique that it will often lessen the pain of a cluster headache.

If, during a migraine attack, the veins appear distended on the forehead or can be seen visibly pulsating, try applying similar pressure over the distended vessels. Almost always, the pain will begin to ease.

☐ Anti-Headache Technique #10: Banish Headaches with This Facial Tone-Up

Poor muscle tone in face and head muscles seems to generalize back into the smooth muscles that surround each blood vessel in the head. Poor muscle tone in blood vessels encourages the constriction and dilation that make headaches possible.

Several headache clinics have found that when voluntary muscles in the face and head are toned up, muscles surrounding blood vessels will assume the same improved tone. As a result, incidence of chronic headache is significantly lessened.

Many people with chronic headaches have reported that, used prophylactically twice a day, this technique has diminished the frequency and severity of both tension and migraine headaches. Still other headache sufferers have found that the same technique has brought speedy relief from a tension or migraine headache that has already begun.

Here's all you do. First, tense your entire scalp, forehead and face muscles, hold tightly for six seconds, and release. Repeat nine more times. Make sure that you tense *every* part of your face, forehead and scalp.

Secondly, raise and lower the eyebrows; squeeze the eyes shut tight, then hold them wide open; wrinkle the nose; make faces; yawn; frown; and wiggle the ears and scalp. Continue these movements for 90 seconds.

Practiced twice a day, this set of action steps promises almost certain prevention and relief for any type of chronic tension or migraine headache.

☐ Anti-Headache Technique #10-A: Morphine for the Mind

Acupressure, or shiatsu massage, is an ancient Oriental method of pain relief that can often stop a minor headache in just a few minutes. Given a little longer, it has been known to subdue the most stubbornly resistant tension or migraine headache.

Scientifically, acupressure has been found to excite small nerve fibers in muscles, causing nerve impulses to be transmitted to the spinal cord and midbrain and on to the pituitary and hypothalamus glands. These glands then release endorphin and enkephalin, the neurotransmitters mentioned earlier that work like morphine to block incoming pain impulses in the spinal cord, creating a natural analgesic.

While acupressure won't remove the underlying cause of headache pain, it often provides startling relief. All you do is apply gentle but steady pressure on certain "pressure points" on the body using the balls of the tips of both thumbs, or sometimes the fingers. While applying pressure, you also use thumbs or fingers to provide a rotating massage. Pressure is usually applied for 7 to 15 seconds, then withdrawn. You can return and repeat the massage a few minutes later. And you can give any number of acupressure applications. Frequently, however, two or three applications are all that is required.

Be extremely careful not to use the nails. Women with long nails may be unable to perform acupressure or any other type of massage. Naturally, you can also use acupressure on anyone else.

These are the principal points favored by acupressurists for headache relief.

1. By far the most popular. is the Hoku Point, the fleshy web between forefinger and thumb on each hand. Place the fingers inside the hand with the thumb on the outside of the web. Using the thumb to press and massage, work around the middle part of the web.

Experience has shown that a single 15-second application here can relieve most minor headaches. By repeating every few minutes over a half-hour period, a persistent tension or migraine headache may disappear. Hoku point massage seems most effective in relieving tension headaches or migraines that center in the eye.

Most acupressurists recommend alternate massaging of hoku points in both left and right hands. However, if the pain is focused on the left side of the head, they will usually massage the left hand twice as often as the right. And vice versa.

Hoku point massage isn't one hundred percent effective. But at each application, the pain usually eases until finally it fades completely away.

2. Gently pinch the lower part of each earlobe and maintain a circular massaging motion.

3. Pinch the bridge of the nose between finger and thumb of one hand and massage. Stay far away from the eyes or eye sockets.

4. Bend the wrist of one hand at a right angle. With the thumb of the other hand, press and massage the side of the arm facing you approximately half an inch above the bend of the wrist. Work around and massage this entire area. Repeat on the other wrist.

5. Clasp the hands on top of the head, with fingertips meeting over the crown. Using the thumbs, massage the hollow in back of the neck, at the base of the skull and level with the ears. Press and massage all around this area.

6. Press and massage the temple areas down to the level of the eyes. Stay on the flat, bony side of the face and stay far away from the eyes or eye sockets.

7. For a tension headache, gently press and massage the points at the hinge of the jaw just below the ears on each side.

8. Using the tips of the forefingers, gently massage the hollow area underneath each earlobe. Remember, we said *gently*.

9. Locate the median line running from the crown of the head down to the bridge of the nose. Along this imaginary line, and on each side of the line about one inch parallel to it, are a cluster of headache-relieving acupressure points.

Using three fingers of each hand, begin at the hairline and work up and back towards the crown. Gently press and massage the area along the median line first, applying pressure for only seven seconds at a time. Then move the fingers one inch away from the line. And once again press and massage points all the way from hairline to crown.

From the crown, you can continue to press and massage all along the median line down to the back of the neck. Next, do the same thing along an imaginary line leading from the crown down the scalp to a point in front of the ears. Finally, press and massage along another imaginary line running from earlobe to earlobe around the back of the neck.

Acupressure points on the scalp tend to be about one inch apart.

10. Place the hands on the back of the skull with fingertips touching. Use the thumbs to press and massage points on the outer side of the neck muscles all the way from the base of the skull to the bottom of the neck. Using acupressure on this area often provides fast relief from tension headaches.

11. Massaging the feet to stop a headache sounds like reaching the attic through the basement door. Yet the feet bristle with nerve endings that respond well to acupressure-type massage. When acupressure is used on the feet, it is known as reflexology. In reflexology, however, both thumbs are used together, side by side, to press and maintain a circular massaging motion on one foot at a time.

Nor is pressing and massaging the feet limited to 15-second bouts. One may continue to massage the feet for as long as desired. After massaging one foot, the other foot is usually given the same treatment.

For headache relief, begin by pressing and massaging both sides of each big toe, then massage the fleshy underside of each big toe. Give these areas a thorough working over. If you feel any tender spots, concentrate on these points. They are often the key to headache relief.

Move next to the area between the big and second toes. Migraines often respond to repeated reflexology massage in this area.

Finally, massage the middle toe of each foot, focusing on the tip. If a headache is located on one side, massage this toe on that side twice as much as on the other foot.

☐ Anti-Headache Technique #11: Brush and Massage Your Headache Away

Since biophysicist Harry C. Ehrmantraut, Ph.D. perfected the technique of the brush massage, thousands of headache victims have made the happy discovery that they can brush their headaches away.

All you need is a natural fiber brush with moderately stiff bristles. Rotate the brush in small half-inch circles so that when you brush the scalp, the upper part of the circle goes towards the back of the head.

Begin brushing above one eyebrow and, rotating in small circles, work gradually back around the temple and dip down the side of the face to below the ear. Continue up again in front of the ear, back and over the top of the ear, and on down the neck.

This pattern takes your brush along both the temporal and occipital arteries. Repeat, starting and staying one inch above the previous pattern. Keep repeating and moving an inch higher each time until you finally brush right back over the center and top of the head and down the back of the neck. Then repeat the whole thing on the other side of the head. With practice, the entire process need not take more than 90 seconds.

The circular brushing motion appears to stimulate both muscles and arteries throughout the scalp and neck, improving muscle tone so that blood vessels return swiftly to normal size. Lacking a brush, you may massage with your fingers, using the same circular motion and following the same patterns. However, when using the fingertips, each stroke should be repeated twice.

Should a headache appear, begin the brushing technique immediately for speedy relief. It appears to work equally well for tension and migraine headaches. After brushing, relief may take a few minutes to appear. You can repeat the brushing technique at short intervals. But be careful not to make your scalp sore.

Professor Ehrmantraut has also recommended doing the brushing technique two to three times a day as a prophylactic measure. The most important times to brush are morning and night. Giving yourself a 90-second scalp brushing on awakening is a wonderfully stimulating way to greet the day.

A few tips: the scalp must be dry. Make sure you brush down in front of the ears, and also on the bony protuberances behind the ears. These protuberances are often a key point in the relief of tension headaches.

If you feel a headache approaching when at a social event, or a meeting or at work, it is usually possible to excuse yourself, go to the bathroom, and give yourself a 90-second brush massage. Most types of women's hairstyles will permit all or most of the headache strokes. However, some migraine sufferers have reported that during attacks, their scalp has become so exquisitely sensitive that they have been unable to brush it at all.

It is vitally important to use a moderately stiff natural fiber brush. For more details, we recommend reading Professor Ehrmantraut's book *Headaches, the Drugless Way to Lasting Relief* (Celestial Arts, 1987).

All in all, brushing is probably one of the easiest and most successful natural ways to overcome headaches.

☐ Anti-Headache Technique #12: Temperature Therapy for Speedy Relief

Before the discovery of aspirin in 1889, the application of heat or cold ranked among the most effective means of treating headaches. While it does take more time and effort than popping a pill, such modern aids as gel packs, heating pads and hot and cold showers have made temperature therapy even more effective today.

Temperature therapy works on three levels. First, heat is used to dilate arteries during the Stage 2 constriction phase in the headache process, while cold is used to constrict arteries during the Stage 3 dilation phase. Second, heat relaxes tense neck and shoulder muscles that initiate tension headaches. Heat followed by a short period of cold is an even more effective muscle relaxant.

Third, applying heat or cold to any part of the body creates what is known as a counterstimulation effect. For example, if we apply the heat to our hands, our awareness shifts from the headache to the sensation of warmth in the hands. In the process, pain impulses from the headache are short-circuited and we become less sensitive to the headache pain.

Never expose your skin or scalp to any temperature that is obviously too hot or too cold for comfort. If you feel uncomfortable, adjust the temperature immediately. And avoid standing under a shower cold enough to shock or cause shivering. A cool, brisk shower is just as effective. Temperature therapy should be pleasant, comfortable and relaxing at all times.

Elderly people, in particular, are advised to avoid exposure to extremes of temperature. And those with diabetes, or other dysfunctions that distort temperature awareness, should have their physician's approval before using temperature therapy. In fact, unless you are obviously fit, hardy and in perfect health, you should check with your physician before adopting any temperature therapy. Naturally, if you are taking a prescription medication or are under medical treatment for any reason, you should have your doctor's approval before using temperature therapy.

Here, in brief review form, are the most effective ways to use temperature therapy for headache relief.

• *Warming the Scalp.* If you can apply warmth to the scalp at the first hint of an impending migraine, the headache can often be aborted. Even if it materializes, after applying heat, the headache is usually mild and subdued.

Many female migraineurs have discovered the advantages of using a bonnet-type hair dryer. They have been largely displaced by the blower type, but can still be found. And countless millions remain stowed away in attics. If you cannot locate one, ask around among your women friends.

Although bonnet-type hair dryers have been used almost exclusively by women, they work just as well for male migraineurs.

At the first sign of an impending headache, set the dryer to "warm" and sit under it. Some women find the warmth so soothing that they often snooze for as long as half an hour. When they wake up, the headache is gone.

As you have probably guessed, the warm air dilates constricted arteries in the head during Stage 2, and the migraine sequence is broken.

Lacking a hair dryer, you could use a hot towel. Dip a medium-sized towel in hot water at not above 112°F (or at a temperature that will not burn your hands or scalp). Wring it out and wrap it in a single layer of another dry towel. Then arrange it on top of the head so that as much of the scalp as possible is covered. Renew every five minutes to maintain temperature.

If preferred, you could try a heating pad set on "low." But moist heat seems to work better.

After several applications, use your fingers to massage your scalp. Using a rhythmic pattern, work right down to the ears and down the back of the neck.

Whether using a hair dryer or towel, stop immediately if you begin to experience actual headache pain—a signal that the headache has entered Stage 3. It's then too late for any more heat therapy. Heat is beneficial only during Stage 2.

• *Stopping a Tension Headache the Lazy Man's Way.* With your upper garments removed, drape a hot, moist towel over the back of the neck and down over the shoulders, covering the shoulder blades and shoulder muscles. Then recline in a deep armchair. Drop the head forward and place the fingertips of both hands on the back of the neck. Lastly, allow the head to fall loosely back.

Using your fingers, begin to massage the neck muscles on both sides of the spine. Work up and down the entire length of the neck.

In many cases, a few minutes of massage will make even the most painful tension headache disappear. If not, renew the towel and give yourself another massage. Even if you have to repeat it a second time, this technique usually stops the average headache in less time than two aspirin.

• *Shower Away Your Headache Pain.* Another speedy way to relieve a tension headache is this. Stand under a warm-to-hot shower and allow the water to flow down over your neck, shoulders and back for at least five minutes. When you feel completely soothed and relaxed, switch to several minutes of cool-to-brisk water. Try and run the water as cool as possible without provoking shock or discomfort, and do not run it for more than four minutes at most.

This technique should release all the pent-up tension in cramped neck and shoulder muscles. By the time you have towelled yourself dry, your tension headache may have completely disappeared. The method is even more effective if you can massage your neck and shoulder muscles while under the shower—or have someone else massage them for you.

Some migraineurs report using this technique to abort an impending migraine attack. For this to succeed, you must begin to shower at the first hint of an aura, or of an approaching common migraine. Play the warm water on your scalp, forehead and neck. For migraine, it is not necessary to cool off with a brisk cold water shower afterwards. Should migraine headache pain appear while showering, stop at once and towel yourself dry.

• *Warming the Hands and Feet*. Warming the hands and feet by immersing them in very warm water is an effective way to end a migraine attack. It can abort a migraine in Stage 2 or it can squelch a migraine headache that has already begun. In fact, warming the hands and feet with water temporarily accomplishes the same effect as does biofeedback (Technique #15). The difference is that warming the extremities in water is a temporary expedient, while the effects of biofeedback are much longer-lasting.

To get started, you need a small footbath or bucket just large enough to immerse both feet above the ankles. Place the footbath so that, while seated, you can also immerse both hands above the wrists in a washbasin or bucket.

For both hands and feet, most people seem to prefer a water temperature just above 110°F. Keep a hot faucet running slowly so that every five minutes you can swiftly refill both the hand and foot baths to maintain temperature.

As the warm water dilates blood vessels in both hands and feet, blood flow to the extremities will increase. This draws blood away from bloated arteries in the head and into the hands and feet. As a result, pressure on arteries in the head decreases and the arteries gradually return to normal size. Within 15 or 20 minutes, many migraine headaches will have been aborted or greatly diminished.

The warmth also stimulates nerve endings in hands and feet which creates a counterstimulation effect in the brain. According to reports from headache clinics, hand and feet warming works well for at least 50 percent of migraine sufferers.

• *Soaking in a Hot Tub.* For tension headaches only, a long hot soak in a tub bath can work wonders in relaxing taut neck and shoulder muscles. It's even more effective if you can stretch your neck, shoulder and jaw muscles for a few minutes beforehand. Raise, lower and rotate the shoulders; swing the arms backwards, forwards and sideways a few times; rotate and loosen up the neck; and yawn several times. Another good tip is to scent the bath with peppermint oil and also to rub some on your temples. This aromatic has a particularly soothing effect that helps ease taut neck and shoulder muscles. While soaking in the tub, it's also helpful to sip a glass of fruit juice.

After toweling yourself dry, lie down and place a cold, damp washcloth, or a cold gel pack, over the headache area. Within a few minutes, all traces of the average tension headache should have completely disappeared.

• *Help for a Sinus Headache.* Experience has shown that steam and moist heat can soothe and benefit a sinus headache. A steam vaporizer works best. But the next best thing is to sit in a bathroom with a spray of steaming hot water running from the shower.

Meanwhile, dip a towel in hot water (not exceeding 112°F), wring it out and cover it with a single layer of dry towel. Then place it across the top of the face and forehead so that it also covers the painful sinus area behind the nose and cheekbones. Reapply the towel every few minutes to maintain the temperature.

After 20 minutes of this treatment, most sinus headaches may be either greatly subdued, or have disappeared altogether.

☐ Anti-Headache Technique #12-A: Using Cold to Kill a Headache

In 1986, a study on ice pack therapy was made at the Diamond Headache Clinic in Chicago. Ninety patients took part, all of whom suffered from acute headaches, including migraine. Half the group used their regular medication for two headaches, after which they used medication plus a cold pack for their next two headaches. The other half used nothing for the first two headaches, and cold packs for their next two headaches.

The overall conclusion was that, when using cold packs, 52 percent of the patients felt an immediate decrease in pain, while 71 percent of all patients and 80 percent of those with migraine felt that cold packs significantly speeded up relief from headache pain. The study showed that while a cold pack is not a panacea, this old-fashioned remedy can still be tremendously helpful for anyone anxious to avoid the side effects of drugs.

Modern gel packs, sold over the counter in virtually every drug store, have replaced the cumbersome ice bag, and have made cold pack treatment available in seconds. Gel packs reduce scalp temperature more rapidly than ice bags and they never melt. However, a plastic bag filled with crushed or broken ice cubes can be used in a pinch.

Cold pack treatment should be used only after headache pain has actually been experienced. It should not be used in Stage 2, that is, during the aura or other warning signs of an impending migraine attack.

Keep your gel packs in the freezer compartment of a refrigerator. To use, cover the gel pack with a single layer of thin washcloth and place over the painful headache area. For migraine, gel packs are particularly effective if placed over large, swollen arteries in the temple. Otherwise, place the gel pack against the forehead.

Most people usually experience pain relief within a few minutes. However, it's best to keep the gel pack in place for at least half-an-hour, by which time the pain should be thoroughly numbed and artery diameter restored to normal.

Naturally, you should sit or lie down while using the pack. A gel pack or ice bag should not be used for longer than 45 minutes at any one time.

Physical therapies are a form of behavioral medicine with important psychological benefits. Using them forces you to take an active role in your own recovery. In turn, this dispels thoughts of helplessness or depression. And your disappearing headaches confirm that taking control of your life and health really does work.

8 The Relaxation Approach

Deep Relaxation is the preliminary step to biofeedback training and to use of creative imagery. Deep relaxation alone has proved enormously successful in relieving and preventing all forms of muscular contraction headaches as well as in aborting classic migraine. Biofeedback is most effective against migraine, and creative imagery is widely used to relieve all forms of headache pain.

Together, relaxation, biofeedback and imagery are the most widely used and successful therapies employed by headache clinics.

DEEP RELAXATION

Almost any type of headache will improve if you can relax. That's because relaxation releases endorphins, the natural narcotics that block pain receptors in the brain and send the pain threshold soaring.

As explained in Chapter 1, the majority of headaches are believed to be caused by emotional stress, particularly by anxiety and depression which trigger the fight-or-flight response, sending the body into an emergency state. It follows that the best way to reduce headache is to stay in the opposite state, one of mental calm and deep physical relaxation.

Practicing deep relaxation with muscle tensing is an important form of behavioral medicine. It requires that you assume an active role in your own recovery and it creates a wonderful feeling of being in control and of being on the path to freedom from medication.

An overall assessment of success rates at a sampling of pain and headache clinics showed recently that relaxation training helped approximately 60 percent of chronic headache sufferers to reduce and control their pain enough so that they could resume a normal life. Most people studied were able to reduce their pain level by 70 percent, though not all achieved total relief. In many people, the regular practice of deep relaxation alone made further pain medication unnecessary. While relaxation does not cure the underlying source of headaches, it is certainly one of the most helpful coping techniques.

Relaxation, biofeedback and pain relief imagery are all akin to self-hypnosis. Among their many benefits is relief of chronic muscle tension. This unnecessary tension not only creates tension headaches but keeps shoulder, neck and jaw muscles tightly constricted, constantly draining energy during much of the day.

Surveys based on a simple muscle-tensing relaxation technique at Columbia Presbyterian Medical Center in New York City found that it provided symptomatic relief for 80 percent of patients suffering from chronic tension headache. Although relaxation appears to benefit tension headaches most, it has also helped relieve the pain of TMJ and combination headaches, and to a lesser extent classic and common migraines.

What Is Relaxation?

During a 1986 study at the Menninger Foundation, researchers Joseph Sargent, M.D. and Patricia Solbach, Ph.D. found that many of their patients were unaware of what it felt like to be deeply relaxed. Only after undergoing relaxation training could they appreciate the difference between tense and relaxed states. One reason is that millions of headache sufferers live in a continual state of emergency and may not have experienced genuine relaxation in many years.

Biofeedback therapists have shown that mind and body are intimately linked. When body muscles are tense, the mind is anxious and disturbed. Conversely, when body muscles are relaxed, the mind also becomes calm and relaxed—a transformation which takes only two or three minutes. And when the mind is relaxed, muscular tension also swiftly drops away.

Important physiological changes occur as we achieve the relaxation response. The breathing rate slows from an average 15–22 breaths per minute to only 4–8 breaths per minute. The pulse rate slows, the mind becomes clear and calm, and every muscle, bone and cell feels completely rejuvenated. We sink into a pleasant state of calm and stillness, liberated from all involvement with anything external.

A caution: because muscle-tensing calls for a brief but strenuous physical effort, anyone suffering from any form of chronic disease, or who is under medical treatment, or who for any other reason should not undertake muscle-tensing, should consult his or her physician before attempting any form of muscle-tension therapy. If you are in this category, you'll want to know that it is possible to skip the physical act of muscle-tensing and still achieve a relatively deep level of relaxation. Muscle-tensing is just faster and more thorough.

Identifying Muscular Tension

To achieve deep relaxation, we must first learn to recognize exactly how tension feels. To do this, lie comfortably on a bed, couch or floor with arms extended slightly from the sides.

Raise your right arm about six inches, make a fist, and tense the entire lower arm from elbow to fist. Tense as tightly as you can and hold it.

Now become aware of the very uncomfortable feeling in your right arm and hand as you hold it under tension. Hold the tension for only six seconds. Then release and gently drop the arm. Note how good it feels as your right arm and hand experience immediate relaxation.

Without waiting, repeat the same tension routine using the left arm. As you hold the left arm tense, compare how it feels with the now-relaxed right arm. Hold your left arm tightly tensed for six seconds. Then release and gently drop it.

No longer should you have any difficulty in identifying muscular tension. Now place your awareness on the face and jaw.

Does your jaw ache with tension? Many tension headache sufferers experience such constant tension in the jaw that it sets up a constant ache in the temples. Constant frowning can also cause a chronic ache in the forehead.

Mentally work over your forehead, eyes, face, jaw and neck, sensing out and identifying tense areas. Most of us can probably identify tension around the eyes. Much of this tension stems from anxiety. But it often becomes so habitual that it continues even after the anxiety has gone.

☐ Anti-Headache Technique #13: Quick Relief for Tension Headaches

A simple tension-relieving technique, originally developed at Columbia Presbyterian Medical Center, may provide swift relief for most tension headaches, and also for some migraines—usually within a few minutes.

Stand erect with feet slightly apart and continue to breathe normally throughout the exercise. Begin by clenching both fists and tensing both arms and hands from the shoulders down. Hold tightly for six seconds. Then release.

Without waiting, tense both legs and feet, including the buttocks. Curl the toes if you can. Hold the tension tightly for six seconds. Then release.

In the same way, tense and release the abdomen muscles . . . the chest muscles . . . and the shoulder and neck muscles. Then screw the face up tightly, press the tongue against the teeth, tense for six seconds, and release.

Now, beginning once more with the arms and ending with the face, repeat the entire process twice more. Finally, do several neck rolls. Shrug the shoulders several times and roll them around. Raise the neck up and push the shoulders down. Then relax. Without holding the breath or stopping at any point, take ten long, deep continuous breaths. Each time you exhale, visualize the pain leaving your head.

If you prefer, you can do the exercise lying down. Although the whole thing usually takes less than three minutes, you can speed it up by tensing every muscle in the body and face at the same time. Hold it for six seconds, then release. Repeat three times before doing the neck rolls and deep breathing.

☐ Anti-Headache Technique #14: Deep Relaxation with Muscle Tensing

More thorough than the previous method, this technique takes you into deeper levels of relaxation from which you can continue straight on into Biofeedback or Creative Imagery. It is an essential preliminary to Techniques #15 and #16.

Choose a quiet room where you will not be disturbed and unplug the phone. Lie down on a comfortable bed, couch or floor rug with a low pillow under the head. Begin by frowning and looking upwards. Hold for six seconds and release.

Press the tongue against the front teeth and squeeze all of the face tightly together. Hold for six seconds and release.

Press the back of the head down on the pillow so that you raise the neck and shoulders off the bed or floor. Hold six seconds and release. Roll the neck loosely from side to side several times.

Tense the neck and shoulder muscles as tightly as possible. Hold six seconds and release. Tense the chest muscles as tightly as you can. Hold six seconds and release.

Raise the right arm six inches off the bed or floor and clench the fist. Tense as tightly as possible from the shoulder down. Hold for six seconds and release. Do the same with the left arm.

Tense the abdomen muscles tightly. Hold for six seconds and release. Tense both buttocks tightly. Hold six seconds and release.

Raise the right leg six inches off bed or floor, curl the toes, and tense the entire leg and foot as tightly as you can. Hold for six seconds, release and lower the leg. Repeat with the left leg.

Next, take five slow, deep breaths, filling the abdomen as well as the upper chest each time. Then resume normal breathing.

Stay relaxed. Place the awareness on the soles of the feet. Silently say to yourself, "My feet feel relaxed. Relaxation is filling my feet. My feet are deeply relaxed. Relaxation is filling my legs. My lower legs are limp and relaxed. Relaxation is filling my thighs. My thighs feel limp and relaxed."

You don't have to repeat these exact words. But give yourself essentially the same suggestions. As you mentally relax each body part, place your awareness on that area and visualize it as limp and relaxed. For example, you might picture your thighs filled with cotton and as limp and relaxed as a piece of tired, old rope.

Continue telling yourself, "My buttocks feel limp and relaxed. My buttocks feel as if they are filled with cotton. My abdomen is limp and relaxed. My shoulders and neck are limp and relaxed. My arms and hands are limp and relaxed. My whole body feels as limp and relaxed as a rag doll."

If you locate any area of tension, mentally relax it before going on.

Now place the awareness on the face as you say, "My forehead feels smooth and relaxed. My scalp is relaxed. My eyes are quiet. My eyes are deeply relaxed. My face is soft and relaxed. My tongue is relaxed. My mouth is relaxed. My jaw is slack."

Be especially watchful for any areas of tension in the eyes, temple or jaw. Repeat these suggestions, as you visualize these areas filled with cotton, until the tension subsides.

Finally, tell yourself, "My entire body and mind are deeply relaxed. I am in a state of deep relaxation."

GOING DEEPER AND DEEPER INTO RELAXATION

By now, your breathing should have slowed and you should be taking slow, relaxed breaths. You can now deepen your relaxation like this.

Picture yourself in a beautiful garden facing a deep, transparent spring. So clear is the water that you can plainly see the white sandy bottom a hundred feet below.

In your imagination, toss a shiny new dime into the

spring. Then, from a distance of about two feet, watch the dime as it darts and rolls and flashes and twists on its slow, silent way to the bottom. Continue to watch the dime closely as it goes down and down, deeper and deeper. After about a minute, it comes to rest on the white sandy bottom. Here in the depths of the spring, far from freeways and telephones, deadlines and pressures, all is completely calm, peaceful, relaxed and still.

Tell yourself once more, "My mind and body are deeply relaxed. I am completely at peace and in harmony with the world. In my mind, I feel only peace, love and joy. I am thoroughly content and completely at ease."

At this point, your mind should feel wonderfully clear and receptive and you should be awake and aware of everything that is going on. Although you may doze off, try to remain awake if possible. Let go of the future and the past, keep your awareness in the here and now, and continue to enjoy every moment.

You can continue to rest and enjoy your deeply relaxed state, or you can continue straight on into Technique #15, Biofeedback, or #16, Creative Imagery. Both are described in the next few pages.

Whenever you wish to return to normal consciousness, remain lying down for a few moments while you open your eyes and move them around, wrinkle and unwrinkle the face, and move each muscle of the body in turn. Then sit up and move around some more. It's best to avoid getting up suddenly.

Making deep relaxation even easier to achieve are a variety of audio relaxation tapes widely advertised in health and New Age magazines. Among the best is *The Relaxation Tape*, recently available for $9 postpaid (possibly higher by now, check before sending any money), from the National Headache Foundation, 5252 North Western Avenue, Chicago IL 60625 (1-800-843-2256, in Illinois 1-800-523-8858).

BIOFEEDBACK

Known in headache clinics by such terms as "Vascular Relaxation through Temperature Biofeedback," this self-regulation technique has shown a high success rate in aborting migraine and in preventing both migraine and tension headaches.

Biofeedback training comes well recommended. Originally developed during the 1960s by Elmer Green, Ph.D. and other pioneers at the Menninger Foundation in Topeka, Kansas, it has since been elaborated on and endorsed by researchers at the Mayo Clinic, Johns Hopkins and just about all of the top university medical schools. Biofeedback training is widely available and its success as a headache treatment and stress-managing technique is unquestioned.

In some situations, professional biofeedback training may be available at quite affordable cost. If it is, by all means take it. Or if your doctor prescribes biofeedback training, you must attend the professional biofeedback clinic that he recommends.

Biofeedback clinics are equipped with supersensitive, state-of-the-art monitoring devices, and with their trained instructors, they can obviously produce swifter results than you can hope to achieve on your own. The snag is that biofeedback training can typically cost from $350 to $1,000 or more for a few sessions of training.

Yet if there is no medical urgency, anyone with some self-motivation and commitment can easily achieve almost equal results with do-it-yourself biofeedback training at home.

Benefits of Biofeedback

A study at Chicago's Diamond Headache Clinic in 1983 reportedly showed that biofeedback helped 70 percent of headache sufferers after other treatments had failed. And a sampling of reports from a variety of headache and pain clinics reveals that after biofeedback training, patients with common migraine have averaged a 75–80 percent reduction in pain, while those with classic migraine achieved a reduction of 85–90 percent. Children as young as eight have been successfully taught to use biofeedback.

Biofeedback works by using your imagination to warm your hands. Tests have revealed that during migraine attacks, hand temperature drops by several degrees. As soon as the attack ends, hand temperature rises again. The temperature drop results from diminished blood supply due to artery constriction. In turn, the constriction is due to a stress mechanism, one of a series involved in the migraine sequence. If hand temperature can be prevented from dropping, the migraine process is unable to continue.

For decades, doctors have regarded hand temperature as an involuntary function over which we have no personal control. But in the 1960s, while studying the benefits of yoga, researchers discovered that we could indeed raise our hand temperature by simply imagining that our hands were heavy and warm.

By making mental pictures, and by giving ourselves silent verbal suggestions, researchers learned that almost anyone can gain voluntary control over hand temperature. That's because the unconscious mind regards all incoming visual and verbal messages as orders to be carried out. A mental picture and a thought are identical, which explains why we must be so careful to think only positive thoughts, and to speak to ourselves only in a positive way. *The unconscious makes sure that we get exactly what we "see" and what we "say."*

Body Talk Counters Pain

As the unconscious receives our mental pictures and verbal suggestions portraying our hands as warm and relaxed, it transforms them into physiological changes in the body. With surprising swiftness, the sympathetic nervous system, which constricts artery muscles, is replaced by the parasympathetic system, which relaxes artery muscles.

Almost immediately, arteries in the hand begin to dilate. As more warm blood flows into the hands, they naturally become warmer and heavier. Even at their first attempt, most people can raise the temperature of their hands by two or three degrees in just a few minutes.

As arteries in the hands dilate, this effect generalizes up the arms and throughout the entire body. The effect is twofold. First, scalp and cranial arteries remain too dilated to enter the Stage 2 constriction phase of the migraine process. Secondly, dilation of blood vessels in the hands and elsewhere draws blood away from the head. This effectively prevents the sudden bloating of arteries with blood should they enter Stage 3 dilation, and the migraine sequence is completely halted.

As we learn to warm the hands and, later on, the feet, we begin to discover that we can gain mastery over our blood pressure, pulse rate, immune system, muscular tension and, indeed, most of the body's other involuntary functions. Thus biofeedback leads to a powerful feeling of self-mastery that quickly extends to other areas of life such as stopping smoking or going on a diet.

So noticeable is this phenomenon that in behavioral medicine it is known as the *enabling effect*. Because all forms of behavioral medicine place responsibility on the patient and involve the patient in playing an active role in recovery, behavioral medicine empowers us to succeed in whatever we do. Compare this with the feeling of helplessness and passivity that invariably accompanies dependency on drug medication.

Do-It-Yourself Monitoring Equipment

Biofeedback clinics have hi-tech equipment that can monitor your pulse rate and blood pressure, muscle tension, skin temperature and brainwave frequency. Seeing these physical functions magnified and displayed on a screen provides a degree of feedback which you cannot hope to match on your own.

Nonetheless, two pieces of monitoring equipment are readily affordable for home use. They are:

1. An electronic digital-readout thermometer that displays the temperature of hands or feet in tenths of a degree.

2. A hand-held GSR (galvanic skin response) device that monitors resistance and displays it as a variable audible tone. Slightly faster than a thermometer, it helps you to learn to relax swiftly.

(We prefer either of these to the adhesive plastic liquid crystal temperature and mood indicators that, though seemingly cheap, have a very short life and a low sensitivity.)

Although not absolutely essential, these inexpensive devices help you recognize the existence of subtle bodily clues by which you can tell whether you are tensed or relaxed. They are often advertised in health or New Age magazines, or can be found in medical equipment stores.

Gradually, as you learn to recognize feedback from your body's signals, these monitoring devices will become unnecessary.

☐ Anti-Headache Technique #15: Overcoming Headaches with Biofeedback

Biofeedback training begins where deep relaxation ends. So the first step is to use Technique #14. With practice, you can soon attain a state of deep relaxation in two or three minutes. Or, if short of time, you could use the faster Technique #13. Either way, let's assume you are lying comfortably in a quiet place with muscles, pulse, lungs and mind all deeply relaxed and with your mind focused on enjoying the present moment and thinking about nothing in particular.

Now begin to imagine yourself in the most restful and pleasant setting you can think of. Childhood scenes often work well. Many people picture themselves sunbathing on a warm, tropical beach. Assuming you use this popular scene, visualize a few flecks of white cloud dotting the wide blue sky, "feel" a gentle breeze caressing the murmuring surf, and "see" the white sails of half a dozen sailboats dotting the aquamarine sea.

Imagine your hands lying on the sunbaked sands. Feel the texture of the sand and, at the same time, experience in your imagination the warmth flowing into your fingers and palms. Use your imagination to experience all the sights, sounds, feelings and smells that go to create this most relaxing scene. As the gulls wheel and cry overhead, "hear" soothing Hawaiian music and "feel" heaviness creeping over your body.

Focus your awareness on your hands and silently repeat these or similar autogenic phrases: "My hands and arms feel heavy and warm. Warmth is flowing into my hands. My hands feel quite warm. My hands and arms are warm and relaxed. I feel my hands glowing and tingling with warmth. My thoughts are relaxed and I am calm and serene. My hands are relaxed and heavy and warm."

And so on.

Images That Heal

By now, everyone is aware that one brain hemisphere is more receptive to verbal input while the other responds best to visual symbols. Feeding both visual and verbal suggestions to the brain saturates the mind with suggestions that your hands become heavy and warm.

Usually, within a minute or two one or both hands will begin to tingle, a sure sign of blood vessel dilation. As soon as you feel a hint of tingling in one hand, mentally magnify this feeling and transfer it to the other hand.

At first, you may find that only one or two fingers on one hand begin to tingle. Don't get discouraged. This is a sure indication that you have achieved a high state of suggestibility, and that the unconscious is carrying out your suggestions. The blood vessels are beginning to dilate in your hands, allowing more blood to flow in to make your hands warmer and heavier, just as you suggested.

Try to notice which mental pictures and suggestions are most effective in making your hand temperature rise. Many people eventually are able to dispense with the beach scene and they end up by directly visualizing warm, fresh blood flowing down their arms and into their hands. They "see" their blood vessels dilate and they "feel" their hands becoming heavier and warmer.

Others have successfully warmed their hands by visualizing them immersed in a bowl of hot water. Still others prefer to picture themselves washing dishes in a tub of hot, soapy water. Yet others imagine themselves reaching out to warm their hands in front of a fire of glowing coals. Use whichever scenes and suggestions work best to warm your hands.

K.O. Your Headache with Biofeedback

Having a digital thermometer or a GSR device enables you to observe subtle increases in temperature or relaxation far smaller than you could unaided. But even without these devices, the fact that your fingers are beginning to tingle is proof positive that you do have mastery over your body. With continued practice, all normal body functions can eventually be brought under your control.

It usually takes 20 minutes to warm your hands on the first attempt. Avoid trying to force anything to happen. Just stay relaxed and continue making the pictures and suggestions.

With continued practice, you can warm your hands in just three or four minutes. After a few weeks, both deep relaxation and biofeedback techniques can be completed in under five minutes. And eventually, many people reach a point at which they can simply close their eyes and imagine that their hands are hot.

If you feel a migraine approaching, lie or sit down, use Technique #13, and continue right on into biofeedback. To assure that the migraine does not return, you may want to repeat it every 30 minutes for two or three hours. Biofeedback is also surprisingly effective in relieving the pain of a migraine that has already begun. And it will enhance the benefits of deep relaxation in relieving and ending muscular contraction headaches.

As a prophylactic against both tension and migraine headaches, biofeedback should be practiced two or three times daily with a gradual reduction to twice and then to only once each day.

Whenever you're ready to return to normal consciousness, open your eyes and move them around, wrinkle your face, roll your neck, and sit up and move around. Then stand up slowly. Your state of deep relaxation and blood vessel dilation should last for at least several hours. Eventually, this condition should become permanent.

If you prefer, you can continue lying relaxed on the floor and go on without a break into creative imagery.

Melodies For Migraine

At the 1986 meeting of the American Psychological Association, psychologist Janet Lapp, Ph.D., of California State University, Fresno, reported the findings of a study which showed that restful or pleasant music could be successfully substituted for the autogenic phrases used in conventional biofeedback training.

By merely listening to popular tunes or to any kind of pleasant, relaxing music, participants in the study actually had fewer migraine headaches, and they could abort a migraine more swiftly than those who used verbal phrases and suggestions.

Listening to music, combined with deep relaxation and visualizing a pleasant scene, is believed to stimulate release of natural endorphin painkillers in the brain. By using music, there is also less need for monitoring equipment. And music also works well for tension headaches.

In another study at Royal Victoria Hospital, Montreal, classical music worked so well as a painkiller that many terminal cancer patients were able to stop taking analgesic medication. Interestingly, the authors of this study found that the more you enjoy a piece of music, the deeper and more slowly you breathe and the more relaxed you become. A tempo close to your heartbeat rate can be very relaxing. Disturbing music like rock 'n' roll is useless. But soothing New Age music, yogic chants, dreamy Hawaiian songs, or classical or popular tunes seem to work well.

If you're interested in taking some of the best biofeedback training available, write: The Menninger Clinic, Box 829, Topeka KS 66601.

CREATIVE IMAGERY

Thirty-two-year-old Jim Bell of West Palm Beach, Florida, had suffered for years from agonizing tension headaches. Only constant medication could deaden the pain. But at the local Wickershaw Counseling Clinic, therapists taught Jim to use his imagination to relieve his pain.

Whenever a headache strikes, Jim lies down and goes into a state of deep relaxation. Then he asks himself what his headache pain feels like. His answer is the first thought that enters his mind.

"My headache feels like a knife plunged through my temple," he may tell himself.

"What would soothe this pain?" he asks himself.

"A block of ice," his mind may reply.

Jim then visualizes a knife plunged deep into his aching temple. On his inner video screen, he "sees" and "feels" the knife being slowly withdrawn from the painful area. As soon as it is withdrawn, he "sees" the upper part of his head encased in a block of ice.

"These images always stop the pain within a few minutes," Jim reports. "The painful area in my head becomes numb. And in fifteen minutes, the headache is completely gone."

Jim is one of thousands of former chronic headache sufferers whose pain has been relieved by a visualization process known as Creative Imagery.

C. Norman Shealy M.D., founder of the Pain and Health Rehabilitation Center, La Crosse, Wisconsin, has stated that he found relaxation and visualization techniques to be the single most important therapy pain clinics can offer to chronically ill individuals with a wide range of problems.

Mind as a Healing Tool

Creative imagery consists of making mental pictures and reinforcing them with silent but strongly positive autogenic phrases or suggestions. By using visual symbols plus verbal affirmations, we create an inner dialog that is immediately understood by both the verbally oriented left brain and the visually oriented right brain.

Our symbols and suggestions are fed through these twin brain hemispheres into the subconscious. Since the subconscious uncritically accepts all symbols and suggestions fed into it, our instructions are immediately relayed to the autonomic nervous system (ANS) to be carried out.

ANS pathways parallel all arterial blood vessels and they control blood vessel diameter. They also control all involuntary body functions from blood pressure to heartbeat and breathing rates, kidney function, immunocompetence, digestion, and production of enzymes and hormones.

By learning to speak the language of the right brain— using symbols and imagery instead of words—our blueprint for wellness is communicated directly through the ANS to the involuntary controls of most bodily functions. And whatever we have visualized and suggested gradually becomes a reality.

Once you have learned deep relaxation, creative imagery is easy to learn and results often come swiftly. At the UCLA Medical School, headache pain was relieved in 60 percent of sufferers the first time they used creative imagery.

Nor do we have to tell the body what to do to relieve headache pain. All we need do is visualize ourselves free of headache, in perfect health, and able to do everything that headaches normally prevent. You don't need to tell the mind how to achieve headache freedom. The subconscious will figure that out at the subclinical level.

Therapeutic Imagery Works Wonders

All you need do is make clear, vivid images and, if possible, "feel," "smell," "hear," and "experience" these images in your mind.

If you do know what actions your body should take, it's fine to visualize this happening. For example, you might visualize the arteries in your head dilating during Stage 2, or constricting during Stage 3. If you aren't sure exactly what arteries look like, symbols are equally effective. You can visualize arteries as a rubber hose, and smooth muscles as fingers clamping down on the hose and restricting the blood flow through it.

Although several popular visualizations are given later, no standard programming exists for creative imagery. You can simply make up your own visualizations and reinforce them with autogenic phrases that best fit the particular headache symptoms you wish to alleviate.

Avoid phrases that use the future tense, such as "My headache will have disappeared by next week." Instead, use the present tense and phrase all suggestions as though your headache had already disappeared.

For example, "The pain in my eye (or temple) has already disappeared. As the ice numbs my headache pain, I feel perfectly comfortable and free of pain. Every vestige of headache pain has already disappeared. I feel very comfortable and at ease."

All phrases must be strongly positive. Avoid negatives such as "I will not," or "don't" or "I won't" or "I will try to." Employ only strong, active, positive phrases and talk as though your headache or other symptoms had already vanished.

Turn On Your Own Placebo Effect

We cannot overemphasize here that your success depends on visualizing yourself as *already free* of headache pain. Pictures and phrases such as "My headache will disappear," make weak, vague instructions to feed to the subconscious. Compare it with "My headache is gone. I am completely free of headache pain."

In a sense, we are mobilizing our own placebo effect. And the key to turning on this self-healing power is a strong belief and implicit trust in the body's own ability to heal itself—a force that we can most easily harness through creative imagery.

For proof, a recent survey of cases of spontaneous remission from terminal cancer found that, without a single exception, every person had possessed a powerful and unswerving belief in his or her ability to recover completely.

We can help reinforce this belief by ending our imagery session with an expression of gratitude for having been healed—even though the healing may not have yet occurred. The vital thing is to "see" ourselves as already healed. Try to feel deeply grateful as you repeat phrases such as, "I am happy and delighted to be free of headache pain. I feel comfort, health and happiness all over my body."

Wind up your imagery session by making strong pictures of yourself already free of headaches and completely recovered. See yourself bicycling through Europe, playing tennis, cross-country skiing or doing whatever it is that your headaches may have prevented.

☐ Anti-Headache Technique #16: Extinguish Pain with Creative Imagery

The first step in creative imagery is to enter deep relaxation (Technique #14). Although not essential, you can deepen this relaxation by adding biofeedback (Technique #15).

You should now be lying down, deeply relaxed. Begin by getting in touch with your headache pain and experiencing it. Exactly where is it? What are its dimensions? Is it constant or pulsating? Can you give it a shape, color, smell or taste?

Then continue with one or more of these frequently-used imagery techniques.

• *Project Your Headache Out of the Body.* Place your awareness on the location of the headache. Visualize its exact shape and dimensions. Now detach this block of pain out of your head and see it several feet in front of you. Meanwhile, visualize a gaping empty space in your head where the pain was formerly located. For instance, you might picture your entire forehead removed from your body.

You can do several things with the painful area you have just detached. You might "see" yourself dropping it into a garbage can. Connect the can to a hot-air balloon and watch it soar away out of sight, never to be seen again.

Or you can visualize the detached painful area out in front of you and fill it with ice-cold water. After it is completely numbed and blue with cold, return it to your head.

Or you can magnify the detached painful area to ten times its original size. Then shrink it down to one-tenth its original size. Repeat this exercise ten times. When back to normal size, fill the painful area with a soothing, bright green light. After a few minutes, return it to your head.

Usually, these exercises so overload the brain with sensory stimulation that pain impulses have difficulty getting through. By the time the exercises are over, the headache has often disappeared.

• *Switch Off the Pain.* Visualize the nerve fiber leading from the painful area in your head to the pain gate in your brain and on to the pain receptors. Just before the fiber enters the pain gate, visualize a large switch operated by an equally large lever. As you experience the headache pain, see yourself pulling down the lever. With a loud clang, you turn off the switch. In many cases, the pain suddenly ends.

As this is a brief visualization, repeat it several times. Eventually, the ANS will turn off the pain gate switch just as you visualized.

• *Displace the Pain.* Focus your awareness on the painful area and briefly experience the pain. Then transfer your awareness, together with the pain, to any other area of your body such as your left foot or right hand. You should feel the pain in this new location, often quite intensely. Meanwhile, the headache area becomes increasingly pain-free.

Repeat several times until almost all of the pain is in the new location. Finally, visualize the pain leaving the new location by flowing out into the air. By this time, the original headache site should be virtually pain-free.

A variation on this is to imagine the headache pain diffused and spread out equally all over the body.

• *Glove Anesthesia.* Visualize one of your hands immersed in an imaginary bucket of hot water. As you maintain this picture, your hand should become quite warm. As soon as you feel this warmth, visualize your other hand plunged into an imaginary bucket of cold water filled with slush ice. In a short time, your hand will feel numbed with cold and it will tingle as if asleep.

Now use this phrase: "I now transfer this numbness to the headache area by touching it with my cold hand." As you repeat this autogenic phrase, place your cold hand against the headache area. Almost everyone experiences a cold, pain-numbing feeling in the head while the headache diminishes.

Repeated several times, this imagery often produces quite dramatic results, even when medication has failed. It is especially effective for migraine relief.

• *Distorting Time.* The rationale behind this popular hypnotic therapy is that time seems to drag endlessly during periods of discomfort while it literally flies during a pleasant experience.

Picture yourself experiencing the most pleasurable sensations you can think of—being given a massage in a luxurious room while beautiful girls bring food and drink—or whatever else arouses sensations of hedonism and deep pleasure. Continue to daydream as you visualize a series of rich pleasures.

As you enjoy the mental feeling, time will begin to fly past just as if you had actually experienced the pleasures you fantasized. And as the passage of time is reversed, so you will find, is your headache pain.

• *Bathing the Painful Area in Sunshine.* Picture a bright ray of healing sunshine flooding the headache area. As you hold this mental picture, repeat autogenic phrases such as these: "My head is entirely free of pain. I feel happy, relaxed and comfortable all over. As the sun's healing rays enter my head, I am completely free of pain. I feel deeply grateful that my inner healing power has restored me to pain-free health."

A few minutes of this imagery usually cuts most headache pain in half. And a few more minutes often ends it completely.

Other Ways to Harness Your Inner Healing Power

Don't forget the technique used by Jim Bell in the opening paragraphs of this section. When using this technique, you can also see your pain as a row of nails driven into your scalp; or you could see your neck muscles tied into knots; or you might visualize your head on fire. As you draw out the nails, untie the neck muscles or extinguish the fire with cold water, your headache diminishes and disappears.

The variety of healing visualizations you can invent is almost endless. You can create images and suggestions to reinforce the effects of any other technique in this book, or to boost the effects of medication or medical treatment.

Creative imagery won't replace such needed therapies as exercise or nutrition, but it can work wonders in reinforcing their benefits. We should also realize that imagery is not a substitute for needed medical treatment. It should not be used to mask pain that has not been medically diagnosed and declared benign.

For best results, you should practice creative imagery three times a day for about fifteen minutes each time. Some people have experienced swift results. In others, it may take several weeks, or possibly longer, for the necessary physiological changes to take place. As new neural pathways and improved behaviors occur, you can gradually reduce the number of daily sessions.

Write Your Headaches Away

Suppose you have trouble making mental images? If so, try writing down your autogenic phrases and suggestions. Enter deep relaxation as usual. Then get up and sit at a table and write down your suggestions. Write them over and over. Writing automatically creates strong mental images of the very suggestions you are writing. Even people with superior imaging ability have obtained still better results by writing.

Since you may get what you "see," it is best not to involve the eyes or other fragile organs in any kind of psycho-technique. Avoid "removing" the eyes from the head or driving an imaginary nail or knife into the eyes. Use an alternative visualization instead.

Imagery techniques should not be used by anyone with any kind of mental instability or mental illness, or who is subject to hallucinations or who, for any other reason, might be adversely affected by using imagery and visualizations. We recommend seeing your doctor before practicing creative imagery.

9 The Positive Approach

Only in recent years have some headache clinics begun to confront the root cause of all headaches, and to stop headaches where they begin, namely in our belief systems. Most appropriately called *cognitive positivism,* this powerful form of behavioral medicine emerged from recent discoveries in immunity research. It was found that the largest single influence on our health and well-being consists of our emotions.

When our emotions are positive, we are able to enter a state of relaxation. We feel calm and relaxed and terrific all over. Our immunity soars and we swiftly become twice as resistant to cancer and all infections. Our arteries relax, our blood pressure drops, and we become virtually immune to heart disease, diabetes, kidney disease and all the other chronic diseases that kill and plague Americans. At the same time, we become almost equally immune to all types of headaches.

When our emotions are negative, we enter the opposite state. We become prone to cancer and infections, our blood pressure rises, and we become increasingly at risk for every type of disease and dysfunction. At the same time, our susceptibility to all types of headaches begins to soar.

The actual process by which inappropriate conditioned beliefs are translated into physiological diseases and into headaches is described in detail under the heading "Stage One" in Chapter 3. This section concludes with the advice that we drop all beliefs that intensify headache pain and replace them with new beliefs that minimize headache pain or that can actually liberate us from headaches altogether.

☐ Anti-Headache Technique #17: Liberate Yourself from Headaches with Cognitive Positivism

Let us begin by restating the psychological axiom that every feeling is triggered in the context of a preceding thought . . . and that each thought that arises is determined by the context of the beliefs that we hold.

Every negative feeling is preceded by a negative thought that arises from holding one or more negative beliefs. Likewise, every positive feeling is preceded by a positive thought that arises from holding one or more positive beliefs.

It doesn't take a genius to figure out that if we drop our negative beliefs and replace them with positive beliefs, we are not only going to have a shot at feeling good all the time, but also that we can become virtually free of headaches and minimize our risk of getting almost any other disease or dysfunction. By changing our beliefs, we change the way we perceive potentially stressful life events.

For example, Smith and Jones are both laid off from their production-line jobs in an outdated plant. Smith fears that he will be unable to find another job. The thought of losing his home, furniture and car, and of being unable to support his family, makes him increasingly anxious and depressed. As Smith continues to perceive the situation in a fearful way, his anxiety increases and he begins to experience frequent tension headaches.

Jones, by contrast, perceives his job loss as a fortunate release from a boring occupation and as a wonderful opportunity to train for a new career in computers. Rather than getting headaches, Jones feels totally confident and capable, an upbeat mindset boosted by secretion of endorphins resulting from his positive feelings.

Although fictional, this illustration is repeated in real life millions of times each day. Both Smith and Jones perceived the same potentially stressful life event. But while Smith perceived unemployment in a negative way that created stress and headaches, Jones perceived his job loss as an opportunity for advancement—a positive viewpoint that left him completely free of both stress and headaches.

When we program the biocomputer that we call the brain with negative beliefs, we get out negative feelings and headaches. When we program it with positive beliefs, we get out positive feelings and freedom from headaches.

If that sounds oversimplified, it's because we are dealing only with cause and effect. The actual bodymind mechanisms involved in the computer analogy are extremely complex. Yet in behavioral medicine, it isn't essential to know *how* the mind or body works—results are what count. And the results we want are the results Jones got.

The big question is: How could Smith change his beliefs so that he too could perceive unemployment in the same stress-free way as Jones?

Healing with the Mind

A key element of the answer is a basic principle of modern psychology—that there are only two root emotions, fear and love. All fear-based feelings are negative, and they include anger, hostility, guilt, resentment, bitterness, frustration, envy, dissatisfaction, anxiety, helplessness, hopelessness and depression. All love-based feelings are positive, and they include joy, peace, generosity, forgiveness, compassion and contentment.

Applying this to Smith and Jones, we see that by viewing life through a filter of fear-based beliefs, Smith perceived a hostile, unfriendly and threatening world. Such a negative way of looking at things intensifies all forms of headache and all types of dysfunctions.

By contrast, Jones viewed life through a filter of love-based beliefs, as a result of which he perceived a friendly, loving and nonthreatening world. Consequently, he remained free of headaches and disease, he felt great, and he continued to enjoy a high level of wellness.

We Can Feel Any Way We Want to Feel

Psychologists have also learned that we can feel any way we want to feel at any time by placing an appropriate thought in our mind. Should a negative thought intrude on our inner video screen, we can easily slide it off. And we can then replace it with a positive visualization, such as a tropical beach scene, before the negative thought has had time to trigger a headache-producing emotion.

In contrast, once a negative emotion has pervaded our consciousness, the strong feelings and upset that it causes can rule us for hours, preventing rational thought and causing us to lash out at people with whom we have close relationships. The result is that we often end up with a tension or migraine headache.

Thinking a thought, incidentally, is the same as creating a mental image, or making a mental picture, or visualizing something. Each of us has complete personal control over our thoughts. For example, close your eyes and visualize a red rose; then picture a snow-capped mountain peak; then a dog.

Were you able to see these objects in your mind's eye? Great! Then this proves that you have the ability to replace thoughts about a rose with alternative thoughts about mountains or dogs. And so it is with negative thoughts that provoke headaches. We can easily slide any negative thought out of our mind and replace it with a more positive thought.

While thoughts can be changed in a split second, it is much more difficult to change a negative feeling.

Think a thought or make a mental picture or visualize an image of a friend or neighbor who has a more exciting spouse, a larger house, a more prestigious job, and a more luxurious car than you do, and you've set yourself up for strong feelings of envy and possibly resentment. Within a few minutes, these negative feelings will start low-level stress mechanisms simmering and you will begin to feel tense, uncomfortable and upset.

Thoughts That Heal

It's not easy to change a strong negative feeling like that once it has begun. But it would have been extremely easy to slide that first thought off your mind when you began comparing yourself with someone else and to replace it with a scene of a beautiful beach. In the process, you could have prevented the unpleasant feeling of envy and continued to feel calm and relaxed.

We must never forget that, at any time, we can personally choose to feel any way we want to feel by placing an appropriate thought on our inner movie screen. Granted, we may have to slide an unwanted thought out of our mind half a dozen times in a row. But by doing so, the mind soon gets the message that negative thoughts are unwelcome. Within a short while, we will find ourselves free of the unwanted thought. And we will also find ourselves free of the headache that the unwanted thought might have triggered.

Learning to control our thoughts isn't really as difficult as most of us believe. Researchers at the University of Pennsylvania and other university medical schools have completely reversed tens of thousands of cases of severe depression by teaching patients to think positively. Called *cognitive therapy*, this method is based on the discovery that many cases of depression are caused not by some complex biological process deep within the body or by the subconscious mind, but by ten easily-recognizable ways in which we distort our thinking by using a negative approach.

Take Charge of Your Headache With Cognitive Positivism

When cognitive therapy is teamed up with positivism, we get *cognitive positivism*, the most powerful healing tool in the entire field of behavioral medicine.

Positivism is simply the opposite of negativity. It implies that we hold only positive beliefs, thoughts and emotions. When we do, we perceive the world in a friendly, nonthreatening way and our minds become calm and relaxed. Swiftly, the hypothalamus recognizes this calm mindset and turns on the Relaxation Response. The entire mind-body enters a calm, relaxed and healthful state in which it remains for as long as we continue to hold a positive mindset.

For as long as we remain in the Relaxation Response, we have no downers or bad moments or bad days and we continue to enjoy every moment of every day. As a result, we experience unbroken high-level wellness and we remain completely free of headaches and other diseases or dysfunctions.

"But I couldn't possibly live like that," you might say. "I need to get angry so I can appreciate the calm periods in between. And how could I feel happy unless I have blue periods to contrast them with?"

If that or something like it was your response, you have probably diagnosed the cause of your headaches.

In reality, the only time we need to experience a fear-based emotion is when we are actually threatened by physical danger. Other "reasons" are all too often excuses by people who prefer the stimulation of strong emotions to the seemingly unexciting alternative of experiencing unbroken calm, joy and inner peace.

There are two easy ways to recognize when we are being run by fear-based beliefs. One is that we may feel too tense and upset to experience calm and relaxation or to use sound, rational, unbiased judgment. Another is that we are coming from a position of scarcity and lack.

When our awareness is guided by fear-based beliefs, we are concerned only with *getting* our own self-interests satisfied. This translates into *getting* security; *getting* enough sex, food and stimulation; and *getting* power through being right or claiming territory or manipulating people; or *getting* more possessions, prestige, fame, recognition, or achievements. On this low level of consciousness—which is where most people spend most of their time—we are primarily concerned with *getting* rather than with giving.

All these positions are based on fear: the fear that there won't be enough to go around; that we won't get our fair share; that our rights may be violated; or that we won't be accorded recognition or prestige. While beliefs on this low level may appear to bring us temporary pleasure, they almost never lead to lasting happiness or satisfaction. All too often they are the cause of chronic headaches.

Worn-Out Beliefs

The headache-causing beliefs we need to let go of are known in psychology as *conditioned* beliefs. Many were picked up in early childhood or in school or in the armed forces or were learned from parents, teachers and other people. Some may have been appropriate in past situations, but the majority are inappropriate to our present lifestyle and they are filling our lives with emotional stress.

These conditioned beliefs based on the past cause us to perceive events in our present lives as stressful. The ultimate way to eliminate the stress that is causing our headaches is to change the way we perceive life events so that we now see them as nonthreatening.

We do that by restructuring our belief system, by letting go of the fear-based beliefs that cause emotional stress, and by adopting new love-based beliefs that liberate us from stress. This type of belief reprogramming can frequently heal chronic headaches in a very short time.

Identifying Fear-Based Beliefs

Most of the headache-causing beliefs we should let go of fit into one of the following patterns.

1. They condemn, judge, criticize or attack someone else.

2. They are unforgiving.

3. They concern the past or future. They cause us to analyze the past and to feel guilt or resentment about something that has already happened. Or they may cause us to worry and become anxious about possible problems that lie in the future.

4. They provoke selfish instincts linked with the body

that arise from fear of lack, and are based on getting and receiving.

5. They cause us to expect a reward for everything we do, or to anticipate fame, wealth, prestige, recognition, praise and other ego-swelling strokes.

6. They cause us to see everything in materialistic terms and to become strongly attached to money and possessions.

7. They cause us to feel discontented and dissatisfied and to crave and want things that are not absolutely essential.

8. They cause us to see difficulties, problems and conflicts in everything.

9. They allow our lives to be run by negative feelings.

10. They confront us with choices when we are tense and emotionally upset. Decisions made when emotionally upset are usually regretted later.

11. They cause us to love a person only if that person meets our conditions.

12. They cause us to compare ourselves with others and to feel dissatisfied.

13. They cause us to compete with and to try to win out over others.

14. They cause us to be rigid and inflexible and to hold strong opinions.

15. They allow us to blame others for the way we are and for what happens to us, creating a convenient victim role for us to play.

16. They cause us to be always concerned with ourselves and to place our own needs ahead of everyone else's.

17. They cause us to fear being alone or doing anything unless we are part of a group.

18. They cause us to magnify molehills into mountains.

19. They cause us to feel insecure, either financially or in relationships.

20. They cause us to feel helpless, hopeless and totally dependent for headache relief on drugs or on passive therapies administered by someone else.

Outdated Beliefs Trigger Destructive Emotions

While beliefs that fit these patterns don't cause headaches directly, they cause us to perceive potentially stressful events in a stressful way.

For example: Julia's sister, acting as executor of their mother's will, keeps for herself a handsome antique clock. Although it wasn't specifically mentioned in the will, Julia feels certain that her mother intended her to have the clock and that her sister was aware of this. As a result, Julia decides that she will never forgive her sister. A few weeks later, she begins to experience migraine headaches. Although she isn't aware of it, whenever she analyzes the past and begins to feel bitter and resentful over the clock, a migraine often appears soon afterwards.

We can easily see that this situation fits into several of the patterns that identify negative beliefs, such as unforgiveness, analyzing the past, wanting things, and so on. Were Julia to let go of these beliefs, in all probability, her migraines would disappear.

To let go of an undesirable belief, you simply *let go of it*. This is made much easier when we replace it with a positive belief. Were Julia to genuinely adopt the positive belief: "I forgive and release forever anyone I have not forgiven, in particular my sister," her migraines would very probably disappear.

Most Headache Sufferers Hold Inappropriate Beliefs

When we continue to hold inappropriate conditioned beliefs—many of them instilled by Madison Avenue brainwashing—we remain locked into a belief system that doesn't work. We spend our time vainly trying to find lasting happiness by buying or doing things which, while they provide a brief glimpse of happiness, only lead in the end to greater dissatisfaction and increasing levels of emotional stress.

Many people believe, for instance, that buying a new car will make them feel happy. It may, for a few days. But then they wake up to the enormous monthly payments they have burdened themselves with and to the huge insurance premiums they must meet. Instead of steering them towards lasting happiness, their negative belief system leads them towards increasing levels of pressure and stress.

A more positive belief system would have steered them towards ceasing to crave a new car. By having their present car repaired instead, they could stay out of debt and remain in a relaxed, positive mind state which would help headache sufferers remain headache-free. Obviously, occasions do arise when a new car, or a new home, may be the soundest investment. But to regard a new car or house as an antidote to unhappiness reveals a serious flaw in a person's belief system.

Positive Beliefs That Liberate Us from Headaches

By adopting the precepts of positivism listed below, we can free ourselves from the majority of headaches.

1. I do and acquire only things which will maintain and deepen my inner peace. I cease craving superficial excitement and stimulation. I realise that lasting happiness comes only from contentment and not from things that I buy, do, eat or drink. When I am content and at ease, my body and mind are calm and relaxed and headaches almost never occur.

2. I forgive and release forever anyone I have not

forgiven—and I rejoice for me. I forgive everyone, everything and every circumstance unconditionally, totally and *right now*!

3. I remain positive all of the time. I accept all the warmth and joy in life but I allow negativity to flow past me and I simply witness it without reacting negatively.

4. I know there is nothing to fear. My headaches will be healed as I let go of fear and as I replace it with unconditional love.

5. I experience only abundance and I am willing to share my abundance with others. For I know that giving and receiving are the same. Whatever I give or lose, I will receive back. (Note: this does not mean you should "loan" money to financially irresponsible people, including members of your own family.)

6. I love everyone unconditionally, including myself, and I accept everyone the way they are without requiring them to change.

7. I am always optimistic, hopeful, cheerful and positive.

8. I completely let go of the past, and with it all guilt and resentment.

9. I have totally ceased to worry about the future. All my fears about the future are imaginary and all my concepts about the future are sheer fantasy. I am a powerful person and I am completely competent to handle whatever the future may bring. Besides, when the future does arrive, it will have become the present.

10. I anticipate tomorrow with enthusiastic expectations. Good things are going to happen to me tomorrow (and also later on today).

11. I live only in the present moment, here and now. Now is the only time there is, for the past is gone and the future is just a fantasy.

12. I choose to enjoy every moment of every day regardless of where I am, what I'm doing, how I'm feeling or who I'm with.

13. I am a hardy person. I am not intimidated by minor discomforts or inconvenience or by physical or mental exertion. I never give up or give in. I always act as if it is impossible to fail.

14. I can heal myself—and I will. I can heal myself from chronic headaches. For healing is to let go of fear and fear-based beliefs. I am completely healed, I can't be sick. Every day in every way I am getting better and better.

15. My birthright is perfect health and perfect health is my normal, natural state.

16. I practice positivism every moment of every day. To be here is joy, to exist is bliss, to be alive is sheer happiness.

17. I act and make choices and decisions only when I am centered, calm and serene. I avoid acting or choosing when I feel emotionally upset.

18. I never use attack thoughts on anyone or anything.

19. I do not expect to be treated with fairness or justice. Both exist only in the eye of a beholder.

20. I accept complete responsibility for my life and for everything that happens to me.

21. I recognize that absolute material security is unattainable. Yet I also know that I will always have what I want when I need it.

22. I always tell the complete truth and I reveal my deepest feelings. I never repress or conceal a negative feeling.

23. I am one with every living thing. I never see myself as separate from others.

24. I always act without anticipating results, without seeking the fruits or rewards of my actions. I act selflessly while expressing love and compassion.

25. I see only the best in everyone including myself.

26. I am content to be wherever I am here and now. I

always have everything I need to enjoy the present moment. Therefore my needs and wants are few.

27. I have no desire for praise, attention, fame or recognition or to appear publicly important. I will not do anything merely to win the approval of others. I refuse to experience pride. I always practice humility.

28. I share the good and success that comes to others without any hint of envy. I never compare myself with others or with their accomplishments or possessions. As a result, I am liberated from envy.

29. I can only win when everyone wins.

Restructuring Your Belief System with Positivism

To put cognitive positivism to work, all you need do is to accept, one by one, each of the 29 positive beliefs. Starting with number 1, study it until you have accepted it completely. Don't go past number 2 until you actually have chosen to forgive everyone whom you believe may have caused you harm at some time.

By the simple act of mentally accepting each positive belief, you will also be releasing its opposite belief, the inappropriate conditioned belief that caused you to perceive events as stressful and that, in turn, caused your headaches.

For example, past events may have conditioned you to believe that the only way to have security is to build a fortress of money. While it may still be prudent to provide for a possible rainy day and for retirement, it is much more appropriate to recognize that life offers an unlimited abundance of love and goodness and that we need no longer continue to look at everything from a position of lack.

Behavioral Medicine's Most Powerful Healing Tool

A rapidly growing body of facts revealed by the leading edge of scientific research is offering intriguing evidence of the mind's healing power. Literally dozens of studies in immunity research are strongly confirming that negative beliefs, thoughts, feelings and attitudes suppress our immunity while positive beliefs, thoughts, emotions and attitudes enhance our immunity. Since our immunocompetence is as closely associated with the fight-or-flight response as our headaches, it follows that the same negative emotions that suppress immunity also cause headaches.

Cognitive positivism evolved out of the pioneering work of such top medical researchers as oncologists Bernie Siegel and O. Carl Simonton, cardiologists Herbert Benson and Dean Ornish, David T. Burns, M.D. of the University of Pennsylvania, Joan Borysenko, Ph.D. of Harvard Medical School's Body-Mind Clinic, Gerald Jampolsky, M.D., originator of attitudinal healing, and Paul Pearsall, Ph.D. of Detroit's Sinai Hospital.

The fact that cognitive positivism has been endorsed by highly accredited doctors from top-ranking university medical schools testifies to its effectiveness. It is the *only* therapy that stops the headache process dead in its tracks before it can even initiate Stage 1. No drug in existence works at this level.

By adopting each of the 29 new positive beliefs, we rid ourselves of negative thoughts. Without a negative thought, we cannot experience a negative feeling. And without a negative feeling we cannot become depressed, fearful, unhappy, angry, anxious, resentful, guilty, or frustrated nor can we experience any kind of downer.

When we deliberately adopt love-based beliefs and thoughts, we begin to see the world as a loving, friendly, non-threatening place. Our focus is on the immediate here and now. By zeroing in on the present moment, we are able to let go of the past and its guilts and resentments, and we realize that whatever the future may hold, we are perfectly capable and confident of being able to handle it.

We begin to see everyone as our brother and sister, and we begin to accept everyone the way they are, and we ask no changes of anyone. We begin to experience a wonderful feeling of oneness with every person and living thing. The concept of feeling separate from other people disappears and with it, any feelings of loneliness.

Right now, at this moment, we realize that there is nothing we need or want. As a result, we feel content and we begin to experience inner peace. We suddenly find we are no longer condemning or judging others. This, then, leads us to forgive everyone whom we once believed had harmed us in some way.

We become almost completely liberated from emotional stress, and from all stress-related diseases and dysfunctions. And somewhere in the process our headaches disappear.

10 The Lifestyle Approach

Headache *prevention* is the theme of the lifestyle approach. And we can achieve headache freedom by assimilating into our lifestyle all behaviors and beliefs that minimize headaches and by dropping all risk factors that intensify headaches.

All too many chronic headache sufferers have built a lifestyle centered around their pain. Gradually, by taking endless medication, they have destroyed their sleep habits, become fearful of physical exertion, developed a poor posture, and acquired habitual use of proven headache triggers, all creating a vicious circle which merely exacerbates headache pain.

We can break this pain-centered lifestyle by taking the first steps towards a headache-free lifestyle. By simply dropping one headache-provoking habit and replacing it with a health-building habit, we can create a powerful change in attitude that immediately motivates us to begin breaking all headache-reinforcing habits.

Most habits, foods, beliefs and migraine triggers that

provoke headaches have been described in earlier chapters. The purpose of this chapter is to review the remainder.

☐ Anti-Headache Technique #18: Live a Headache-Free Lifestyle

Stop Smoking

Not only is smoking a suicidal, health-wrecking habit but it is one of the major causes of all types of headaches. No one can feel completely safe from headaches until he or she has quit smoking for good.

Space prevents our giving a complete stop-smoking strategy. But we do know that more people are addicted to nicotine than to all street and prescription drugs combined, and that smoking is as addictive as heroin or cocaine.

Nicotine stimulates production of beta-endorphin and certain neurotransmitters that cause alertness, arousal, a feeling of pleasure, and freedom from pain and anxiety.

What smokers fail to realize is that regular daily exercise, such as a brisk five-mile walk, provides exactly the same level of alertness, arousal, and a feeling of pleasure, and freedom from pain and anxiety as does smoking, all without the health risks of smoking. (All smokers should have their doctor's permission before taking up exercise.)

Additionally, most stop-smoking authorities advise switching from smoking to chewing a nicotine-based gum like Nicorettes. The goal is then to gradually break your addiction to the gum—a task made much easier when you exercise daily.

You are also advised to enroll in a non-commercial stop smoking clinic sponsored by the American Cancer Society, American Lung Association, American Heart Association or the Seventh-Day Adventists. To complete your program, you should have your doctor issue you an absolute and strongly worded ultimatum to quit smoking immediately.

The many other steps you can take are described in books or are taught in the clinics. Don't be afraid of gaining a few pounds. To equal the health risk of smoking, you would have to be 120 pounds overweight. And if you do slip up, begin to quit smoking again *immediately*. Don't take a second cigarette. A single slip won't wreck your intentions.

Maintain Regular Sleep Patterns

Sleeping with your head under the covers permits an oversupply of carbon dioxide to accumulate in blood vessels. Carbon dioxide is a powerful blood vessel dilator and migraine trigger.

Anyone who sleeps for under five hours or for more than ten hours each night also increases risk of migraine. Fatigue due to lack of sleep is another well-known migraine trigger. Thus it's important to maintain regular sleep patterns throughout the week. Get up at the same time every day and avoid oversleeping on weekend mornings.

Those prone to tension headaches should avoid sleeping on the stomach. It forcibly turns your head to one side, creating muscular tension that could easily set off a headache. If you sleep on your back, place a small pillow beneath the neck to prevent the head from being tilted either backwards or forwards. Likewise, if you sleep on your side, avoid slumping the head forward.

Special "cervical pillows" are available, designed to allow the neck to relax while sleeping on the back or side. You may also obtain a horseshoe-shaped pillow stuffed with a gel pack which you can freeze in the refrigerator and place under the head and neck to relieve a headache. Called the Suboccipital Ice Pillow, it is available from SPF Distributors, 1545 North Verdugo Road, Glendale CA 91208. This mention does not imply our endorsement.

Use Your Diary to Identify Headache Triggers

Careful diary-keeping is a great help in identifying the exact nature of tension or migraine headache triggers. Women should include exact dates on which menstruation begins and ends. After three months, you should begin to see a pattern which can help to identify migraine triggers and to avoid them.

Diary-keeping coupled with careful observation also can help identify tension headache triggers. For example, you may find that it is not typing that causes your headache but the way you sit or slouch over the typewriter. Or it could be due to inadequate lighting. Identifying and avoiding headache triggers has brought relief to many.

Here is a brief rundown of the principal categories of headache triggers.

PHYSICAL AND ENVIRONMENTAL TRIGGERS

Smog-containing sulphur dioxide, commonly emitted from refineries, steel and paper mills or fertilizer plants, has been scientifically confirmed as a common migraine trigger. Fumes and odors from soap, detergent, perfume, after-shave lotion, and household chemicals and pesticides, when inhaled in an enclosed room, can set off migraine in some people.

Other common environmental triggers include glaring or flickering lights or bright outdoor sunshine (wear sunglasses and a hat with a brim).

Stale air in offices and rooms, especially if smoke-filled, is a potential headache trigger. Others include: odorless carbon monoxide leaks from car exhausts or heating equipment; rapid decreases in barometric pressure; wearing a swim mask or goggles—this can set off a headache one to two hours later; sudden weather changes, especially onset of a hot, dry wind.

Loud, jarring noises keep the body continually stressed, while a constant noise prevents relaxation. Temporary headaches due to high elevation are also common among mountain hikers and climbers. Usually mild, the headaches customarily affect the entire head. Occasionally, an altitude headache is confined to one side, and can become as severe as a migraine. Altitude headaches normally disappear on descending.

Long distance flights, especially from east to west, can trigger migraine in susceptible persons. To help avoid headaches when flying, drink frequent glasses of water, avoid alcohol, eat lightly, sit in an aisle seat so that you can stand up and stretch, and rest upon arrival. OTC painkillers are freely available on most flights.

POOR POSTURE TRIGGERS

Abrupt changes of posture can trigger tension headaches. Avoid cradling a phone under your chin for more than a few minutes. Sit up straight and keep the head erect and the shoulders low while using the phone. Whether standing, sitting or lying, keep the shoulders *down*. Avoid hunching them up around the ears.

Avoid slouching or slumping at any time, especially while watching TV. Place the TV screen at the same level as your eyes and straight in front so that you avoid looking down or turning your head. Get up and walk around at least once per hour, roll and rotate the shoulders and neck, and pull the shoulder blades together several times.

Avoid working overhead with your arms and hands raised for long periods. Use a stepladder instead. Don't permit your head to slump or hang forward. Always sit and stand tall, straight and upright. When sitting at a desk or working at a bench, change positions every fifteen minutes. Breathe through the nose, keep your tongue relaxed, and avoid grinding the teeth. Also avoid shallow breathing. Inhale fully and fill the bottoms of your lungs at each breath.

Reading or working in a poor light is a common cause of headaches. Use a bulb with a minimum power of 60 watts directed down over your shoulder. We used a 250-watt soft white light bulb mounted overhead while writing this book. Fluorescent lighting is even better. The older you are, the stronger the light you should have.

Poor posture while slouched over and reading in bed can also contribute to tension headache. Avoid reading in bed with your head propped up on pillows. Instead, sit upright in bed with a pillow under your knees to prevent pressure on muscles in the lower back. Always sleep on a pillow. Sleeping without a pillow causes more blood to flow to the head, setting the stage for a migraine attack.

TIME PRESSURE STRESS AS HEADACHE TRIGGER

People whose lives are filled with deadlines and pressures commonly suffer from tension or migraine headaches. Most of us can slow the pace of our lives by letting go of nonessential activities such as volunteer work, and by turning down all demands on our time that create added pressure.

Almost all of us are able to put the brakes on a busy helter-skelter lifestyle so that we have more time to work, play, eat and relax at a leisurely pace. With careful planning, we can usually rearrange our lives to take time out each day for fun, games and socializing.

Build up a week's income in reserve so that you don't have to stand and wait in line at the bank or supermarket during the Friday afternoon crush. Go on Tuesday instead. Shop early in the morning or after 7 P.M., when supermarkets are often empty. Plan activities well in advance so that you start out in plenty of time, especially for work. Find the location of new places you must visit on a street map before you leave home. And prevent rush by doing only one thing at a time.

Although Americans tend to glorify the automobile, and a car is essential in most locations, driving under today's high-speed conditions is far from pleasant. Several studies have concluded that car ownership actually lowers the quality of most peoples' lives. It places a severe strain on our finances, while driving and maintaining a car can be one of the most stressful aspects of modern living. Among other things, it can entrap us into becoming a chauffeur for our children.

Try to minimize driving on freeways or in congested traffic. For short trips, use a bicycle or walk instead. And you can help reduce automobile stress by keeping your older car instead of buying a new one, and by spending as little time in the car as you can.

Try to avoid a sudden letdown from stress as you end a hectic week on Friday afternoon and find yourself in an inertia vacuum on Saturday morning. This situation can frequently provoke a migraine, especially if your job entails long days of listening, talking, telephoning and making decisions.

The answer is to even out your work week, and to try and spread your tasks and work load evenly over each day. Most of us could gradually phase out a crowded schedule by pacing ourselves differently. Many migraineurs create unnecessary stress by their inability to live with an uncompleted task. The solution, of course, is to never be afraid to postpone completion of a nonessential task.

Above all, we need to learn to live life for today and to enjoy every moment for what it's worth.

NATURAL
COLD REMEDIES

Contents

Acknowledgments

Much of the research on which this book is based was derived from some of America's most eminent university medical centers and from such sources as the National Institutes of Health, the Food and Drug Administration, the National Academy of Sciences and the Public Citizen Health Research Group. Almost all of these studies support the validity and effectiveness of the holistic approach to healing and of the various alternative healing methods described in this book.

So many direct and indirect sources were consulted in researching this book that it is impractical to acknowledge every one. However, I would like to acknowledge my debt to the research carried out by Alan Barreuther Ph. D., assistant professor of pharmacy and advisor to the Self-Care Cold Center, University of Arizona; Benjamin Siegel, Ph. D., professor of pathology, Oregon Health Sciences University; O. Carl Simonton, M.D., of the Simonton Cancer Center; Ananda S. Prasad M.D., Ph. D., professor of medicine, Wayne State University; Dr. Roy Walford, professor of pathology, UCLA; Patricia Wagner, Ph. D., University of Florida; Dr. Robert Henkin, director of the Center for Molecular Nutrition and Sensory Disorders, Georgetown University Medical Center, Washington D.C.; the American Academy of Otolaryngology, Washington D.C.; the Department of Health and Human Services, Food and Drug Administration, Rockland, Md.; and hundreds of other contemporary holistic health pioneers who have taught us that a Whole Person approach is the most essential step in achieving swift recovery from any disease or dysfunction.

1 Conquer Your Cold in Twenty-four Hours

Five hundred million colds beset Americans annually, causing a loss of 46 million workdays, and each winter week 13 percent of the population catches a fresh cold.

Yet the message of this book is that you can easily eliminate 80 percent of the risk that you will catch a cold this winter. And if you do catch a cold, chances are good that you can recover completely not later than the evening of the second day.

Credence for these claims comes from the breathtaking succession of discoveries through which science has already unlocked the secrets of the common cold.

We have already learned the structure and design of cold and flu viruses and the entire process by which viruses enter the nasal passages and replicate themselves in cells lining the mucous membranes.

Because the common cold may be caused by one of over 200 different strains of rhinovirus, or similar virus, science has been unable to produce a vaccine. A new form of alpha interferon spray, which may prevent up to forty percent of colds if used correctly, may soon be approved by the FDA. But despite some pioneering success with monoclonal antibodies and with a drug called WIN 51,711, medical science can still do little more than soothe the symptoms of the common cold.

Much of the newly discovered information about the common cold and flu has emerged as a by-product of cancer research. And most cancer research today is centered on immunology—the study of white blood cells (soldier cells) charged with defending the body against infection and disease.

Both the common cold and flu are caused by viruses which are recognized as foreign invaders and are identified as non-self by the body's white blood cells. Cancer occurs when a body cell's genes go berserk and become so genetically different that the cell, too, is identified as non-self by white blood cells.

Thus both cancer cells, and cold or flu viruses, invoke a similar response by the immune system.

Whether white blood cells can overcome and destroy a cancer cell depends on the overall competence of the body's immune system. When immunocompetence is high, white blood cells are able to destroy each individual cancer cell that appears in the body before it can begin to clone into a tumor. When immunocompetence is low, a cancer cell may survive undetected and divide and grow into a tumor.

Immunocompetence Is Key to Cold Demise

When pitted against cold or flu viruses, the immune system eventually always wins. But the speed with which a person's immune system can wipe out a cold or flu is largely governed by his or her immunocompetence. In viral infections, immunocompetence focuses on the speed at which specialized white cells can manufacture antibodies and other virus-fighting immune system components.

In a person with low immunocompetence, a cold may linger on for ten to fourteen days before the immune system can finally muster sufficient antibodies to destroy it.

In a person with average immunocompetence, a cold typically lasts about seven days. A person with moderately high immunocompetence may be rid of a cold in only four days.

But a person with optimal, peak immunocompetence can often recover from a cold completely within twenty-four hours.

New research is showing that many of the therapies which have been suggested in the past, such as taking vitamin C or zinc gluconate lozenges, are effective boosters of immunocompetence.

Only a Whole-Person Approach Can Bolster Immunocompetence

However, exciting new discoveries are emerging to show that the type of optimal, or peak, immunocompetence that can consistently annihilate a cold in a very brief time can be achieved only by a holistic or whole person approach.

It has been found that three principal factors can enhance immunocompetence. They are: 1. Nutrition and light eating; 2. Regular exercise; 3. Positivism, which translates into thinking positively, staying emotionally calm, and being physically relaxed and free of tension.

While our eating habits, and how we exercise, form an important and essential contribution to bolstering immunocompetence, recent advances in immunological methodology have confirmed that Positivism is the largest single influence on the body's health and well-being.

Put together, Nutrition, Exercise and Positivism interact synergistically so that the sum total of their overall results is many times greater than the cold-fighting power of any one of the three factors considered alone.

This explains the varying results and the controversy which has surrounded such unholistic therapies as taking vitamin C without the support of other essential nutrients, and without the wider support of exercise and Positivism.

When vitamin C therapy is supported by other essential nutrients, and by exercise and Positivism, immunocompetence can be dramatically boosted, often in a matter of hours.

Why Brisk Walking Beats Chicken Broth

At this point, you may be wondering how you are supposed to exercise when you are coming down with a severe cold. Or how you can become totally relaxed and attain a positive, optimistic and hopeful attitude while suffering from a miserable viral infection. Or why you may be asked to chew carrot sticks and sip a rich onion soup liberally garnished with garlic and cayenne pepper instead of more traditional foods such as chicken broth.

You may discover that some of the most cherished cold remedies of the recent past have been exposed as weak and often ineffective. Carrot sticks, for example, supply much needed vitamin A which is essential to the integrity of cells in the nasal air passages as well as to immunocompetence. Likewise, onion soup laced with garlic and cayenne pepper has been found a more effective cold remedy than the traditional chicken broth.

Fats of all types have been identified with low immunocompetence while fresh fruits and vegetables supply nutritional support sorely needed by an overburdened immune system.

Exercise boosts immunocompetence, clears the nasal passages and reduces discomfort from cold symptoms. So, if you feel up to it, a brisk thirty-to-sixty minute walk can do far more for your cold than sitting in front of a TV set. (Obviously, you cannot exercise if you have a fever or if you feel too fatigued.) And both Deep Relaxation and Positivism are easily learned in a matter of minutes while lying in bed.

It is true that you may achieve good results with vitamin C or with zinc gluconate tablets alone. But you can invariably achieve far more satisfactory results in half the time by using a Whole Person approach.

Positive Thinking Is the Best Cold Therapy

It may come as a surprise to learn that thinking positive thoughts and staying physically relaxed can do more to conquer a cold than any other single therapy. But the simple explanation is that stress is unable to exist when we are deeply relaxed and thinking optimistically. Like most other human diseases and dysfunctions, cold and flu are stress-related and they begin to improve almost immediately when we free ourselves from emotional stress and tension.

This book is built around a scientifically-validated explanation of the common cold and flu disease processes. Alternative therapies are suggested only where they integrate with scientifically-proven facts. However, as drug remedies continue to produce adverse side effects, or to prove ineffective, medical science is gradually accepting alternative therapies. For example, Deep Relaxation and Positivism have become the principal tools of that branch of medical science known as Behavioral Medicine. Thus even these very subjective methodologies have been scientifically validated.

While medical science has focused its efforts on destroying the cold virus, or rendering it impotent, most alternative therapies have focused on how severely a cold may affect us. The message of the Whole Person approach to healing is that we *are* able to modify our personal response to a common cold infection. Those who respond best, it has been found, are people with the most relaxed and optimistic attitude and the highest overall level of physical activity and nutrition.

The function of this book is to describe everything you can do to minimize risk of catching a cold or flu; to lessen the severity of cold or flu symptoms should you become infected; to dramatically shorten the duration of any cold or flu you may catch; and to prevent any complication, such as bronchitis, pneumonia or strep throat, from occurring afterwards.

Why Holistic Therapies Work Best

As in every other area of health and healing, a holistic approach is the only system that really works. For example, permanent weight loss is extremely difficult to achieve through dieting alone. Not until exercise and stress management are added, does a diet really begin to work. Likewise, exercise alone will do little to lower cholesterol levels and prevent heart disease until a low-fat diet and a stress management program are added.

In the entire health field, there are remarkably few magic bullets: no anti-aging pill that really works, and very few foods or nutrients that, singly and alone, produce dramatic results.

For a cold therapy to really work, it must work on all levels: on the nutritional, physical, psychological and even the spiritual levels simultaneously.

The chapters in this book are arranged so that you can

begin to practice a step-by-step holistic cold-therapy program as you read. Right at the beginning, Chapter 1 tells what you can do to start treating your cold and to begin feeling better almost immediately.

In a single reading, Chapter 3 makes you an expert on the pathology of the common cold and flu. Not only will you understand every step in the cold process but you will learn to distinguish a cold from the flu and how to tell if more serious complications arise.

Chapter 4 familiarizes you with the drugs and treatments developed by medical science and it explains why modern medicine can still do little more than ease the distress of cold or flu symptoms.

Chapter 5 describes how to boost your immunocompetence with nutritional support. Chapter 6 describes the most effective non-drug cold remedies used by herbalists. Chapter 7 covers the entire spectrum of things you can do physically to bolster immunocompetence. Chapter 8 describes how and what to eat to speed recovery from a cold.

Chapter 9 shows how to achieve peace of mind by thinking positively. Chapter 10 describes another way by which you may achieve peace of mind by deeply relaxing the body and by using creative imagery. Chapter 11 describes how to avoid catching another cold in the future.

If you already have a cold, read Chapter 2 right now and get your holistic therapy started. Then continue to read this book, chapter by chapter, so that you will learn how to continue the therapy you have begun.

In the entire field of holistic healing, the key to success is acquiring the necessary KNOW-HOW. To treat your cold successfully, you must know everything there is to know about the cold process and how to deal with it.

You can acquire the know-how you need in the least possible time by reading carefully right through this book. We suggest you read the following chapters in numerical order. This is not a large book and the average reader can easily complete it in a single evening. If you then put into practice what you have learned, chances are good that your cold should have disappeared by bedtime on the following day.

2 Ten Ways to Fight Your Cold and Start Feeling Better

Suppose you have just come down with a cold. Your nose is stuffed-up and runny. You have a bad case of sniffles and you're sneezing all over. There's an ominous, scratchy feeling in the back of your throat, your nose feels tight, and the skin around your nostrils is already raw and burned. Your eyes are watery and you feel like blowing your stack instead of your nose.

Now that a cold virus has hit you with its double whammy, what can you do right away to start feeling better and to begin the recovery?

Obviously, there isn't time to read right through this book. That's going to take several hours. So here are ten steps you can take that will launch you off on the right track immediately. You may not want to try them all. But taken together, they do offer a Whole Person approach to getting well again.

It's important to realize that the ten steps are a stopgap measure to give you the time to read this book right through.

You should make every effort to read this book completely on the evening of the first day that your cold symptoms appear. The therapy in some of these steps, notably Step Three, should not be continued for more than twenty-four hours until you read Chapter 5 for more detailed information.

The same applies to most of the other steps. To treat a cold intelligently, you must know everything about the cold process and the safe and correct way in which to apply each form of cold therapy.

Otherwise, your "cold" might actually go unrecognized as influenza or another type of upper respiratory tract infection. It's vital to be able to recognize exactly which dysfunction you may be suffering from and to know when to seek medical help if needed. All this information is in Chapter 3. But you *must* read Chapter 3 to understand it. The same rationale applies to every other chapter.

So here they are: ten easy ways you can take to start fighting your cold and to start feeling better, while they buy you the time you need to study the remainder of this book.

Step One: Take a Brisk Walk if You Can, for One Hour or More

Naturally, this advice applies only if you feel up to walking outdoors. You certainly should not walk if you have a fever or the flu or if you feel at all weak or fatigued. However, a brisk walk of three to four miles stimulates the entire immune system. It also accelerates the absorption and metabolism of nutrients essential to immunocompetence.

Continuous rhythmic exercise outdoors opens up the nasal passages and makes breathing easier. And it stimulates production of opiate-like endorphins in the brain that kill the pain and discomfort of cold symptoms.

Alternatively, you may practice any form of continuous rhythmic exercise such as jogging, bicycling, swimming in warm water, or local cross-country skiing. If you pedal a stationary bicycle, try to use it near an open window or on a porch where you can breathe fresh air.

Once the exercise is over, stay indoors and rest and relax for the remainder of the day.

Important Caution: walking or other exercise is suggested only to persons who are already physically fit and healthy, who regularly perform this same exercise at least several times each week, and who are able to walk or exercise without any ill effects. Do not suddenly begin to exercise if you are not already fit and healthy enough to complete the exercise without any risk to your health.

To continue this therapy, read Chapter 7 (under subhead *Exercise Briskly Every Day*).

Step Two: Stop Smoking Completely and Cease Drinking Alcohol for as Long as the Cold Lasts

Both smoking and alcohol seriously impair immunocompetence and increase risk of further viral and bacterial infection. You should also try to cut out coffee and minimize intake of other caffeine-containing beverages such as black or green tea, hot chocolate, cocoa and most cola drinks. However, you may make an exception of an occasional cup of green or black tea with lemon if it makes you feel better.

To continue this therapy, read Chapter 7 (under subhead *Stop Smoking*) and Chapter 8 (under subhead *What Is a Good Anti-Cold Diet?*).

Step Three: Begin Taking
Nutritional Supplements

Many cold sufferers have a deficiency of vitamins A and C and the mineral zinc. Lack of these nutrients hinders production of immune system components needed to destroy invading viruses.

Begin by taking 10,000 IU of vitamin A. If unavailable in supplement form, you could take a tablespoon of cod liver oil followed by consumption of two medium-sized raw carrots. Slice the carrots into sticks and munch them all before bedtime.

Simultaneously, take one gram of vitamin C. Every two and a half hours thereafter, while you are awake, take an additional 500 mg.

Also begin to take one 50 mg. zinc gluconate lozenge every two hours while you are awake. Be careful not to chew or to swallow the lozenge but *allow it to dissolve slowly in the mouth*, a process which may take ten minutes or so.

All of these nutrients are available in health food stores.

To continue this therapy, read Chapter 5 in its entirety. It is important that you read this chapter on the same day that you begin to take the nutrients recommended in Step Three above. Do not continue the vitamin-mineral therapy described above for more than one day until you have read Chapter 5.

Step Four: If You Have a Sore Throat,
Start to Take Slippery Elm Lozenges.

This traditional herbal remedy is available in most health food stores.

To continue this therapy, read Chapter 6 (under subhead *Cough Suppressants*).

Step Five: Drink Plenty of Fluids

Try to drink half a glass of water or other non-alcoholic fluid every half hour throughout the day. This is needed to replace fluids lost during the healing process and by fever.

Hot drinks and soups also act as expectorants by helping loosen secretions from the chest. The one best cold-fighting beverage is considered to be onion soup liberally flavored with garlic and cayenne pepper. Miso broth is also excellent as are unsweetened fruit and vegetable juices, especially orange, grapefruit, apple or grape, and carrot or tomato juice. Ideally, they should be freshly squeezed; fruit juices may be cut with an equal amount of water. Carob drinks and herb teas, especially chamomile, are also recommended. Lemon tea is particularly soothing.

Equally good is this lemon beverage; cut up two lemons and steep in a pot of boiling water for twelve to fifteen minutes. Serve in a cup with a tablespoon of honey and sip slowly.

Alternatively, you can squeeze the juice from a large lemon and mix into a glass of warm water. Sip it slowly. Each of these lemon-based drinks increases the acid level of mucosa in the throat, a condition that helps soothe throat discomfort and also destroys invading viruses.

To continue this therapy, read Chapter 8 (under subhead *Grandma's Remedies* and *Foods That Heal*).

Step Six: Adopt an Anti-Cold Diet and Eat Lightly

Many foods of animal origin plus most fats, and white flour and sweeteners, delay cold recovery. They do so in a variety of ways, ranging from hindering absorption of more essential nutrients to a direct reduction in immunocompetence.

Numerous studies have also linked light eating with increased immunocompetence.

Begin by cutting down drastically on fats, especially hydrogenated vegetable oils and saturated fats. This means eliminating most meat; whole milk dairy products, especially cheese and ice cream; eggs, all fried or fatty foods, and poultry skin from the diet. White flour, sugar and sweeteners of all types (except honey served in beverages) should also be eliminated. Avoid all convenience and fast foods, processed and canned foods, commercial sauces and dressings, and mayonnaise.

Replace them with fresh fruits and vegetables, seeds, nuts, whole grains and legumes. Especially beneficial are carrot sticks and all yellow-orange fruits and vegetables as well as deep-green leafy vegetables. Citrus, and particularly tangerines, are highly recommended. You may also include one tablespoon of either safflower or sunflower oil mixed into your diet; the oil should be cold-pressed.

Once a day, spread a quarter cup of wheat germ on your breakfast cereal or on any other food. And do eat as many foods as possible raw or unheated. Steam, bake and stew instead of frying. Good sources of whole protein are baked fish or plain, low-fat yogurt, low-fat cottage cheese or skim milk.

Take care not to overeat. Large, heavy meals or stuffing of any kind weakens immunocompetence. Eat lightly and only when hungry.

To continue this therapy, read all of Chapter 8.

Step Seven: Increase the Humidity and Clear Your Nose

Humidity keeps the mucous membranes in the nose damp, enabling them to repel invading viruses and to trap and destroy millions of others. If you have a humidifier or vaporizer, use it to humidify the air in your home. Lacking either, turn the thermostat down a couple of degrees and leave a kettle or a pot of water simmering on the stove.

To decongest the nose, mix a teaspoon of salt into a glass of warm water and inhale it through the nose until it runs back into the throat. Blow the nose gently and steadily using disposable tissue. Five inhalations will usually clear the most stubbornly-blocked nostrils.

Next, boil a kettle full of water and pour it into an open dish. Place the dish on a plate or pan and put it on the table. Lean over the dish, keep the eyes closed, cover the head with a towel, and inhale the steam into the nasal passages, sinuses and lungs. The steam swiftly breaks up all congestion and also makes the nose too hot for viruses to thrive.

A *caution:* do not be tempted to inhale steam direct from the spout of a kettle; you may get burned.

To continue this therapy, read Chapter 7 (under subhead *Keep the Mucous Membranes Moist, Inhaling Steam,* and *How to Clear a Blocked Nose*).

Step Eight: Make Yourself Comfortable

Assuming you do *not* have a fever, take a long, relaxing soak in a hot tub bath. If only a shower is available, let the water run as warm as you can stand with comfort, and allow it to flow over the back of your neck and shoulders and on down the back. Do not bathe or shower if you have a fever.

Prepare a cup of green or black tea, or a herb tea, and add a teaspoon of lemon juice. Sip it as you relax in bed. Then settle down comfortably and read the remainder of this book. Or read something else you enjoy.

Don't get up until you are certain you do not have the flu or a fever (see Chapter 3 under subhead *How to Tell*

Whether You Have a Cold or Influenza). Rest in bed for as long as your temperature remains above normal.

To continue this therapy, read Chapter 7 (under subhead *How to Feel Comfortable Quickly*).

Step Nine: Stay Calm and Relaxed

Numerous experiments have demonstrated that immunocompetence soars when the body is deeply relaxed and the mind is calm and serene. In controlled studies, a measurable rise in immunocompetence has occurred in as short a time as one hour.

Ideally, this step should follow Step Eight and you should be lying in bed sipping a cup of hot tea with lemon and perusing the pages of this book. If not, remove your shoes and tight clothing and lie down flat on your back. Keep the arms and legs flat and support the head with a pillow.

Take six long, slow deep breaths. Take care to fill the bottom of the lungs first, before expanding into the top. Gradually slow the rate of breathing to four breaths per minute. Complete twelve or more long, slow, deep breaths.

Then, limb by limb, mentally relax your entire body. Relax each arm and each leg, the shoulders and torso. Then relax the forehead, eyes, cheeks, mouth, tongue, jaw and neck. Picture yourself as relaxed as a rag doll or a string puppet.

Now, imagine yourself in an elevator at the top floor of a 100-story building. Look up at the floor indicator above the door. It now displays the digital number 100. The elevator then begins to descend at a rate of approximately one floor every two seconds. Keep watching the indicator as it counts down the floor numbers from 100 to 1. Silently count along with the indicator as you look up at it.

By the time you reach the ground floor, you should be in a delicious state of detachment from worry and pressure, with every muscle free of tension and with the mind calm and unruffled.

To continue this therapy, read Chapter 10 up to and including the subhead *How Biofeedback Can Help Shorten Your Cold.*

Step Ten: Think Positively

Thinking positive thoughts, called Positivism, has been scientifically validated as having more influence on the body's health and well-being than any other factor. It bolsters immunocompetence even more than does relaxation. Thinking and being positive can do more to shorten your cold and reduce the severity of symptoms than anything else.

Ideally, thinking positively follows completion of Step Nine.

To get started, make a mental picture of yourself in the most relaxed and worry-free spot that you can think of. Most of us will probably choose a beautiful park or garden scene or the countryside or a tropical beach. Picture it vividly, in full color with a wide blue sky overhead flecked by white tufts of cloud and a light breeze caressing the rakish coconut trees that line the shore. Absorb every detail of this pleasant scene as you lie in the warm sun on the grass or beach. Notice that you are feeling terrific: cheerful, optimistic, friendly and hopeful.

Now, whenever a negative thought crosses your mind, slide it off your inner movie screen and replace it with the restful beach or garden scene you have just created. You don't have to hold the beautiful scene in your mind permanently. But you do now have something with which to immediately replace a negative thought should one occur.

From now on, refuse to entertain a negative thought. This means you will be automatically free of all negative feelings. No negative emotion can occur unless it is first triggered by a negative thought. By refusing to allow a negative thought to persist on your inner movie screen, you can only feel upbeat, optimistic, hopeful and loving.

Pause now and ask yourself if there is anyone you feel resentful or angry about or envious of. If so, forgive them completely, now and forever, for any harm you believe they may have caused you at any time.

Whenever any thought about the past enters your mind and you experience resentment or guilt, slide that thought out of your mind and replace it with the beach or garden scene.

Likewise, should any thought regarding the future produce anxiety or worry, slide that thought off your inner movie screen and replace it with the beach or garden scene.

This simple technique will eliminate all resentment, guilt, worry or anxiety. Keep your awareness centered in the present moment and completely let go of the past and the future.

Enjoy being in the present moment, even if your cold symptoms do seem rather distressing. Feel grateful that you are warm and safe and in a comfortable place with good music, books, videotapes, health-building foods, juices and hot soups, and everything else you have reason to be thankful for.

As you let go of the past and future, you will find it easier to stop judging and condemning others. And as you focus on being in the here and now, you will realize that you already have everything you need to enjoy the present moment.

As a result, you can stop wanting anything and begin

to experience contentment. Contentment, in turn, leads directly to peace of mind.

Immunocompetence is maximized only when we have complete peace of mind. And inner peace can occur only when the body is relaxed and we have released all negative beliefs, thoughts and feelings.

To continue this therapy, read Chapter 9 in its entirety.

3 The Anatomy of a Cold

It was a Friday afternoon in mid-February and Bob Rhinehart, a thirty-five-year-old Florida real estate salesman, was on his way to a closing party. The gathering was to honor Jack Fetterman, another salesman who had just closed an important deal.

Bob greeted Jack with a hearty handshake.

"How's it feel to make five grand in a day?" Bob asked, as he picked up a chicken drumstick and began gnawing on it.

"Oh, the money's great, of course," Jack answered. "But I think I'm coming down with something. My nose feels dry and tight. There's a scratchy sensation in my throat. And somehow I don't feel quite up to par."

Jack's surmise proved correct. He spent the weekend at home nursing one of the most virulent colds he'd ever experienced. To avoid giving his cold to others, Jack also stayed home on Monday. But despite Jack's good intentions, it was already too late. The common cold becomes contagious almost a day before any symptoms actually appear.

Moments before Jack and Bob shook hands, Jack had touched his nose. When he shook hands with Bob, ten million microscopic cold viruses were transferred to Bob's hand. A moment later, Bob had touched his face as he gnawed on the drumstick. This move placed at least eight million invisible cold viruses at the entrance to his nostrils.

What happened next reads like a science fiction Cell Wars drama. A breathtaking succession of recent discoveries in the science of immunology has revealed that there's a lot more to the common cold than a sore throat and a runny nose.

As five million viral invaders burst into his nose, Bob's body became a battleground for an invisible yet incredibly complex war between his body's white blood cells and the legions of invading viruses.

More than a week was to pass before Bob's defenses were finally able to rout the penetrating micro-organisms and emerge victorious. It was this desperate but unseen life and death battle within his own body that created all of Bob's distressing cold symptoms: the perpetually runny nose, the endless sniffles, the bouts of sneezing, the raw, burned skin around the nostrils and, later in the week, the sore throat and the loss of his voice.

Massive Viral Invasion Penetrates Our Defenses

Within minutes of arriving, most of the viruses were inhaled into Bob's nostrils. Many were immediately trapped, like flies on a flypaper, by the wet, sticky mucosa lining his nasal passages. Legions of cilia—whiplike hairs beating continuously in unison at 600 sweeps per minute—then pushed these trapped invaders steadily toward Bob's gullet and down his digestive tract to be destroyed by stomach acids.

But about half the invaders managed to evade the beating cilia. They lodged against some of the millions of body cells lining Bob's nasal passages.

Immediately, Bob's nasal cells sensed the presence of a hostile invader and they began to signal for help. They did so by releasing microscopic amounts of a prostaglandin— a hormone-like substance—into the bloodstream. This particular prostaglandin serves as an emergency chemical messenger to alert the immune system. Within minutes, all nearby macrophages and helper T cells began to head for Bob's nasal passages.

Consisting of a mere 600 atoms, and so small it can be detected only in an electron microscope, a virus is nothing more than a bundle of genes encapsulated in a protein coat. While not actually alive or able to move, a virus exists in a twilight zone between the largest complex carbon molecules and the smallest mammalian cells.

The rhinovirus is the type most frequently responsible for the common cold. Over 120 varieties of cold-precipitating rhinoviruses have been identified, which explains why a cold vaccine has never been produced. The rhinovirus is shaped like a geodesic dome, composed of twenty triangular-shaped surface facets. This tough micro-organism possesses the unique ability to shuffle the amino acids in its protein coat so that its twenty surfaces are constantly changing their antigens (cellular fingerprints).

Masters of Subversion

An antigen is also the surface receptor at which the host's immune system directs its missile-like antibodies.

Another cunning strategy developed by the rhinovirus has been to place these receptors in a deep, hard-to-reach cleft on each of its twenty facets. These subterfuges allow the rhinovirus to trick its way past the vigilantes of the body's immune system—the powerful macrophage cells. Like sentinels eternally on watch, these large scavenger cells roam the nasal blood vessels, as well as every other blood vessel in the body, on a constant surveillance mission. Whenever they encounter an organism with a non-self antigen, they zero in for the kill.

The immune system is the body's defense organization against infections and cancer. Essentially, it consists of one trillion white blood cells, each of which is totally dedicated to destroying all non-self cells and particles in the body, whether living or not. Once recognized as non-self, organic invaders like cold or flu viruses are immediately attacked by the full range of the immune response. Whether fungus, protozoa, bacteria, virus, multicelled organisms or our own cancer cells (which become non-self), all are relentlessly attacked until either the immune system or the invader wins out.

As the surviving rhinoviruses fanned out and contacted the cells in Bob's nasal passages, some of the viruses were recognized as non-self by roving macrophages. But the viruses so outnumbered the macrophages that only a few were caught.

Nevertheless, each macrophage within range closed in on a virus. Then, using its arm-like pseudopods, the macrophages groped deep within the clefts on the viruses' surfaces. Some were able to pluck out a viral antigen.

This triumphant act effectively sealed the virus's fate. From now on, these captured antigens would serve as patterns for the manufacture of billions of antibodies. In a few days or a week hordes of antibodies would paralyze and destroy the unwelcome virus.

The Body Fights Back

Swiftly, then, each macrophage displayed a virus antigen on its own surface next to one of its own antigens. Patrolling the nasal blood vessels were a few helper T cells, white blood cells programmed to "read" viral antigens. Quickly, these helper T cells binded with receptors on the macrophages. Once a helper T cell had scrutinized both the self and non-self antigens on its surface, each macrophage released the lymphokine interleukin 1. Each helper T cells then became activated.

Upon becoming activated, each helper T cell began releasing a variety of lymphokines, chemical messengers that alerted every component in Bob's immune system and identified the target. The activated helper T cells first released interleukin 2, a growth factor which increases production of additional activated helper and killer T cells and also stimulates the activity of macrophages. They then released the lymphokine "B Cell Group Factor" which triggered B cells to multiply. B cells are another type of white cell whose function is to mass-produce antibodies.

Activated helper T cells next released gamma interferon, a stimulant that makes killer T cells more aggressive, that summons more macrophages to the target site, and that urges B cells to produce more antibodies. Finally, the activated helper T cells released "B Cell Differentiation Factor", a lymphokine which instructs most B cells to eventually stop replicating and begin antibody production.

This constant interchange of lymphokines between the immune system's various components orchestrated and amplified their attack. The most urgent task was to produce whole new armies of white blood cells. Each lymphocyte (a collective name for T and B cells) can divide and multiply into 500 new cells within four days. Macrophages and similar scavenger cells can divide and multiply into thirty-two cells within six hours.

Nutritional Deficiencies
Cause Defenses to Falter

But such a massive build-up is possible only when sufficient amounts of zinc and other nutrients are on hand and when immunocompetence is high. The competence of our immune system in destroying invaders is a reflection of our own physical and mental health. When we exercise regularly, eat lots of fruits and vegetables, and have a positive, upbeat and hopeful attitude, our immunocompetence is enhanced.

Had Bob's lifestyle been built around such factors, his immune system might have conquered the cold in just a day or two. Unfortunately, Bob had been recently divorced. He seldom exercised any more. He lived largely on hamburgers, coffee and fast foods. And he often experienced bouts of lingering depression. As a result, his immunocompetence was so suppressed that his cold lingered on for twelve misery-filled days before his immune system was finally able to erase it.

Regardless of how competent is one's immune system, however, the same step-by-step conflict occurs as in Bob's case. The only difference is the speed at which the body girds itself and fights back. A person with really high immunocompetence may be able to throw off a cold by the second day.

But no matter how high one's immunocompetence, in the beginning the immune system is largely unprepared and helpless to stop the tidal wave of beseiging viruses. Millions of rhinoviruses were now in contact with the cells lining Bob's nasal passages. Most were able to bind on to receptors in the host cell's wall.

In response to the pressure on its surface, each cell puckered up around the virus and—possibly believing it to be a nutrient—innocently absorbed the micro-organism into its cytoplasm. In the process, each host cell released an enzyme that removed the virus's protein coat. This left the virus core exposed, a tiny piece of translucent RNA (ribonucleic acid) containing its genetic code for reproduction.

Triumphant Virus Proliferates

Once a virus hijacks a cell in this way, it shuts down the cell's own genetic software and the virus's genetic software takes over. In response to this new programming, the cell then begins to turn out between 100 and 1,000 clones of the virus's genetic package. Included in the viral genes are instructions for the cell to re-encapsulate each new virus core in a protein coat.

While all this was going on, Bob's infected nasal cells were desperately trying to warn neighboring cells. They did so by releasing interferon, another lymphokine. As this interferon touched each nearby cell, that cell became incapable of replicating viruses. Unfortunately, the interferon was insufficient in amount to reach all of the cells in Bob's nasal passages. Tens of millions remained unprotected.

C DAY MINUS ONE

Twenty-four hours after the viruses first arrived, Bob was still unaware of the lonely battle being fought in his body. He had no cold symptoms and he still felt fine.

But by now, at least a million cells in his nasal passages had been commandeered by viruses and transformed into virus factories. Some cells already contained as many as a thousand copies of the original virus invader

As these newly-manufactured viruses drifted close to the outer wall of infected cells, they were detected as non-self by activated T cells. Teaming up, lymphocytes and macrophages attacked the hemorrhaging nasal cells. But as each cell burst open, releasing up to a thousand more viruses, the lymphocytes were overwhelmed. Floating along on the breath nearly a billion new viruses began to migrate all over Bob's upper respiratory passages, penetrating his sinuses, the Eustachian tubes that led to his ears, and working down to his tonsils, adenoids, and throat. Meanwhile, infected cells that had hemorrhaged began dying in droves. To prevent blood loss, the immune system sent fibrinogen, a clotting agent, to dry up the blood in Bob's nasal membranes.

We Become Contagious Before Cold Symptoms Appear

At this point, still without any cold symptoms as yet, Bob became contagious. As had happened with his friend Jack Fetterman the day before, should he touch his nose and then touch someone else's hand or face, the probability was high that he would transmit some of his own rhinoviruses on to that person.

Although Bob wasn't yet coughing or sneezing, he could expel millions of viruses into the air with a strong exhalation. Traveling on invisible molecules of water vapor floating in the air, these viruses could then be inhaled by other people. Thus, while the majority of colds are transmitted by hand-to-hand contact, or by touching an object recently handled by a cold victim, colds may also be caught by inhaling air in a room occupied by someone infected with a cold virus. Complicating the task of preventing colds is that someone can be contagious while still free of all cold symptoms.

Thus far, virus production had far outstripped the manufacture of white cells by Bob's immune system. For every virus destroyed by killer T cells and macrophages, a hundred thousand more were ready to replace it.

By now, however, some of Bob's B cells were ready to commence antibody manufacture. Dwelling unseen in the lymph nodes and spleen, B cells are able to produce thousands of antibodies in a single minute. But gearing up for this kind of production *can* take up to several days in a person with poor immunocompetence. And before antibody production can commence, the B cells must examine a sample of the virus antigen. Hence, one of the tasks of helper T cells was to carry a viral antigen to each B cell cluster. The B cells then produce antibodies which are a mirror image of the virus antigen.

How Armies of Antibodies Zap Cold Virus

Antibodies are thus able to lock onto the viruses' antigens, hampering their travel, making them functionally impotent, and marking them as targets for phagocytes (large white cells which devour foreign matter).

Although reinforcements of killer T cells and macrophages were by now hastening to Bob's nose, the viral enemy was so enormous that only antibodies could finish them off.

Hence it is the speed of antibody production that will govern the duration of Bob's cold and the severity of his symptoms. Once antibody production catches up with the number of viruses, the viral invaders are doomed.

But antibodies are complex particles. They can be produced only when B cells are adequately supplied with minerals and other essential nutrients, the source of which is Bob's diet. Indications are that antibody production is significantly speeded up when a plentiful supply of zinc and vitamins A and C are available in the body.

COLD DAY

Forty-eight hours after the first viruses arrived, at least half the healthy cells in Bob's nasal passages had been infected. As millions of dead and dying cells accumulated in his nose, nasal tissues start to secrete histamine which boosts blood flow to the nose and causes swelling and congestion. In turn, this stimulates mucous membranes to produce copious amounts of mucus to wash away the dead viruses and cells. Inflammation is, therefore, a natural defense mechanism which plays an essential role in the immune response.

As these changes gradually took place, Bob became vaguely aware of an oncoming cold. He felt a mild but scratchy tickling sensation in his throat. His nose and throat seemed dry. He lost his usual hearty appetite and felt mildly fatigued. And as the day wore on, it became all too apparent that a bad cold was approaching. By evening, both his nostrils were completely blocked while mucus flowed like water. Bob experienced bouts of uncontrollable sneezing. His eyes began to water and he had a mild headache. He felt tired, feverish and completely miserable.

C DAY PLUS ONE

After a fitful night, Bob woke feeling thoroughly uncomfortable. As did hundreds of others in his city that day, Bob called in sick, took two aspirin, drank plenty of fluids and stayed in bed.

What Bob and most others failed to realize is that cold symptoms, uncomfortable as they seem, are a clear indication that the body is taking strong measures to heal itself.

What we call a cold is really the symptoms of a healing process. Bob's ceaselessly runny nose was his body's defense against further viral invasion. The inflammation in his nasal passages was part of his body's immune response to contain the spread of infection. Unfortunately, the swollen tissue and free-flowing fluids exerted pressure on nerve endings and caused him unceasing pain and discomfort.

Fever is also an occasional cold symptom designed to kill viruses. Most cold and flu viruses have been living for thousands of years in the air passages of the human organism at a temperature slightly below that of the body's normal core level of 98.6°F. These viruses are extremely sensitive to temperature change. In its efforts to destroy viruses, the body raises its core temperature to as high as 104°F.

This rise of several degrees is enough to immobilize billions of cold and flu viruses as well as many other pathological organiams. Fever, then, is a natural body response to get rid of invading viruses. You can shorten the duration of any infection by allowing the body to maintain its fever and by avoiding the use of any medication or aspirin to lower your temperature. Unless your temperature is really excessive (104°F or over) a fever is a sign that your body is basically healthy and is responding to an infection. (However, temperatures of 104°F or over are usually high enough to require immediate medical care.)

Although the common cold can lead to complications, by itself it is almost never fatal. Eventually, even the weakest among us muster sufficient antibodies to ensure its demise. Technically, the common cold is considered a self-limiting, upper respiratory tract infection and in most people it clears up spontaneously in under fourteen days.

However, in some people it is stopped dead in its tracks by the second or third day. What makes the difference is our immunocompetence.

C DAY PLUS TWO

Although aspirin dulled his discomfort, none of the various over-the-counter preparations Bob took affected the course of his cold. Deep within his body, billions of white cells toiled to speed up antibody production. But Bob's mediocre level of immunocompetence hampered their efforts. Without adequate levels of zinc and other essential nutrients, his immune system took eight days to accomplish what a person with a more competent immune system might have achieved in a single day.

C DAY PLUS THREE

Today, Bob managed to drag himself out of bed. Despite the misery he was enduring, he forced himself to go to work.

C DAY PLUS FOUR

His constantly stuffed-up nose caused Bob to breathe through his mouth. No longer was the air he inhaled cleansed, warmed and moistened by his nasal cilia and mucous membranes. An endless post-nasal drip also irritated his throat.

C DAY PLUS FIVE

On this day, the viruses were able to infect the vocal cords in Bob's larynx. His voice became a mere croak and he was constantly hoarse. However, in his upper air passages, for the first time in a week, viral production began to taper off, due primarily to a shortage of remaining cells to infect.

C DAY PLUS SIX

While Bob's immune system still struggled with anti-body production, he became almost voiceless and his larynx felt swollen and tender to the touch. Bob felt even more depressed than usual and he was unable to relax.

C DAY PLUS SEVEN

After waiting for essential minerals and other nutrients to gradually filter through from Bob's nutrient-deficient diet, his immune system finally managed to produce the required antibodies.

Antibodies belong to a class of proteins called immunoglobulins. Most of the antibodies manufactured by Bob's B cells were Type M immunoglobulins. Intended only for temporary use against his present cold, they would fade away a few days after the cold was overcome. However, some of Bob's B cells were producing Type IgG immunoglobulins, a more permanent antibody that would live for several years, or even for a lifetime. Should Bob ever catch a cold of this same virus strain again, these antibodies would stop the infection on the spot.

Sweeping through his lymph and bloodstreams, vast populations of antibodies poured on to the virus hordes still occupying the nasal passages. Locking on to antigen receptors on each of the billions of viruses, the antibodies began to activate a series of enzymes known as complement. Together, the antibodies and complement neutralized the viruses. They also served as markers for millions of larger phagocytes, white cells which literally swallow viruses and digest them.

C DAY PLUS EIGHT

The full impact of Bob's immune system was now unleashed on the viral invaders. Antibodies, complement, phagocytes, killer T cells and macrophages, all attacked the viruses in unison.

Like other immune system components, complement production had also been slowed by Bob's poor diet and his other counterproductive lifestyle habits. Defects in his complement system contributed significantly to his susceptibility to laryngitis.

C DAY PLUS NINE

As the viruses in Bob's nasal passages began to thin out, his head cold showed signs of improvement. But he was still plagued by hoarseness and a painfully sore throat. He felt tired and depressed.

C DAY PLUS TEN

Although his nasal cold symptoms had begun to clear up, Bob's voicelessness and sore throat were still so uncomfortable that he had difficulty in sleeping.

C DAY PLUS ELEVEN

For the first time in nearly two weeks, Bob was able to

breathe through his nose again. But his sore throat and laryngitis lingered on.

C DAY PLUS TWELVE

On this day, Bob's immune system completely vanquished the last of the viruses in his nose. Bob's head felt fine again. But it was another twelve hours before all of the viruses in his larynx and throat were destroyed.

C DAY PLUS THIRTEEN

Now that the viruses were gone, Bob's bloodstream was filled with rampaging hordes of killer T cells, macrophages and antibodies, all on the lookout for trouble. Thirsting for blood and almost out of control, these aggressive immune-system components can mass in joints such as the elbow or knee and once there, attack the body's own cells. This situation is known as auto-immunity and rheumatoid arthritis is the most common of the many dysfunctions it can cause.

Auto-immunity usually seems to occur only when the immune system's suppressor T cells are weakened by severe and prolonged emotional stress. Normally, as in Bob's case, suppressor T cells take over control of the immune system at this stage. Sending commands by lymphokines, they turned off all B cell antibody production and halted further attacks by killer T cells. Under their urging, Bob's entire immune system gradually slowed to non-combatant status.

Only phagocytes were permitted to continue cruising in the nasal area to mop up the debris. Within a few days, most of the lymphocytes and antibodies replicated for the conflict had died off. But some lymphocytes would live on in Bob's bloodstream for several years or more. Each would remain sensitive to the antigen of the specific virus which had produced Bob's cold. And as long as these lymphocytes lived, Bob would be immune to that specific rhinovirus.

As we experience cold after cold during a lifetime, we gradually do acquire immunity to an increasing number of cold viruses. This phenomenon explains why children aged one to three often catch one cold after another, as do young schoolchildren. During these early years, the body is exposed to a continual series of new cold viruses to which no prior immunity has been developed.

Gradually, as we grow older, we acquire immunity to an increasing number of common cold viruses. As a result, colds gradually become less common with increasing age.

INFLUENZA

Influenza is another viral disease that follows a similar pattern to the common cold. After initial exposure to flu virus, it takes two to three days for influenza symptoms to appear. Most cases of flu are spread by airborne transmission during the three days following the first appearance of symptoms. However, many victims remain contagious for several additional days.

Influenza symptoms appear more swiftly than do cold symptoms and they strike with greater severity. Unlike a cold, which is localized in the upper respiratory tract area, influenza is a more widespread disease with considerable potential for serious complications.

Almost without warning, a well person is suddenly struck by shivering and chill, body aches and pains, a headache, extreme fatigue and a fever with temperatures ranging over 101°F in adults and as high as 104° in children.

The spherical flu virus contains a genetic package similar to that of a cold virus. But its protein coat is also covered with fat and studded by spikes. To outwit patrolling macrophages, flu virus populations undergo a constant change of antigens induced by a gradual but steady mutational drift.

As the human population builds up antibodies to a flu outbreak, the mainstream flu virus is annihilated. Only mutants with different antigens are able to survive. These mutants then multiply to become the mainstream flu virus.

Nonetheless, their antigens still so resemble those of the earlier strain that they are partially affected by antibodies left over from the last flu infection. As a result, new strains of influenza resulting from mutational drift are relatively mild. They rarely present a serious threat to healthy adults or children and medical treatment is seldom required.

Every so often, a strain of flu virus seems to disappear from the human population. Some researchers speculate that it may spend several years submerged in animals such as swine or ferrets. While in the animal kingdom, this virus undergoes a spontaneous mutational shift so radical that its antigens become completely immune to all existing human antibodies.

Defenders Caught Unprepared

When it resurfaces in man, the human immune system is caught completely unprepared and a sudden, widespread epidemic occurs. The Spanish Flu pandemic of 1918 was the worst pestilence to afflict the human race. Over half a million died in the U.S., and thirty million more elsewhere on this planet. Another 50,000 died in 1957 when Asian Flu hit the U.S. and infected 45 million Americans.

Scientists have identified three types of influenza virus.

•TYPE A is the most frequent and severe. Its subtypes are also the most subject to variation. Type A variants have been responsible for almost every major pandemic, including the Spanish Flu of 1918, the Asian Flu of 1957 and the Hong Kong Flu of 1968. Type A variants continue to cause flu epidemics every two to three years and it is the most common flu type encountered in the U.S. during winter.

•TYPE B causes local flu outbreaks, especially in spring or summer. Because it is less subject to variations, there are no important subtypes. However, Type B viruses do experience mutational drifts that can cause devastating new strains to appear every few years.

•TYPE C is rarely encountered nowadays.

Variants of each type are named for the major surface protein and for the proteins that induce immune response against the virus. The two major proteins are hemagglutinin ("H") and neuraminidase ("N"). Thus H1N1 is a recent subtype that was identified in Chile in 1981, while H3N2 surfaced in the Philippines in 1983.

Although by itself flu is a self-limiting ailment and is rarely fatal, complications present a potentially serious risk to the elderly, the chronically ill and to some pregnant women; to those with chronic lung diseases such as tuberculosis, asthma, bronchitis and emphysema; or to patients with diabetes, heart disease, kidney disorders, cystic fibrositis or obesity.

As with the common cold, the severity and duration of influenza appears related to the victim's immunocompetence. A person with a strong immune system may recover from flu in only four or five days while the infection can persist for ten days or more in a person with a compromised immune system.

In, say, a forty-year-old adult with an average immune system, fever typically lasts three days, after which symptoms gradually ameliorate. However, even though you may suddenly feel well, it's advisable to schedule an extra day of rest at home in case of a relapse.

Although influenza is responsible for a whole catalog of miseries, one thing it does *not* cause is so-called "intestinal flu." This term is commonly used to describe a variety of gastrointestinal ailments, such as persistent indigestion, nausea, and diarrhea, which people believe are caused by a flu-like virus. However, the comparison is inaccurate. Neither flu nor cold viruses produce any kind of gastrointestinal dysfunction nor are these problems related to the aftermath of a cold or flu.

HOW TO TELL WHETHER YOU HAVE A COLD OR INFLUENZA

Without taking a lab test for antibody titer, no physician can positively identify whether you have a cold or flu. And the test takes so long to culture out that the dysfunction could be nearly over before the answer was known. Hence doctors rely on physical symptoms to diagnose an upper respiratory tract infection.

The symptoms are often so clear that you can make a fairly accurate diagnosis yourself.

Cold Symptoms

Cold symptoms appear rather gradually and tend to be localized in the nasal area, spreading later down to the throat and larynx or bronchial tubes. The most common cold symptoms are a scratchy throat and sneezing, sniffles, watery eyes, and a stuffed-up, runny nose. Fever is not common in adults and is usually slight. A sore throat, a mild cough, and viral laryngitis, hoarseness or voicelessness may occur during later stages. A cold may cause a higher fever in children but high temperatures are rare in adults. A mild headache may occur. Symptoms actually experienced depend on the specific virus causing the infection.

Influenza Symptoms

By comparison, the onset of flu symptoms are more sudden and severe. Fever may quickly soar to the 102° to 104°F range. Headaches are common and prolonged. Muscular aches and pains appear throughout the body. A sore throat is a frequent symptom. Bouts of chill and shivering often alternate between periods of sweating. The eyes are sore, the face is often flushed, and the skin hot and moist. The victim feels weak and fatigued and appetite may fade. Almost 90 percent of flu victims are afflicted with dry, hacking cough and, often, a chest discomfort also. Existence of a local flu epidemic supports the probability that the diagnosis of influenza is correct.

Alarming as they may appear, flu symptoms pose little risk to a healthy adult or child. In any case, medical science is unable to cure or alleviate either a common cold or flu since antibiotics are ineffective against viruses.

Because both cold and flu viruses may create raw, irritated tissue, and also overload the immune system, a bacterial infection of the nose, sinuses, throat or chest may follow a cold or flu.

Danger Signals of Serious Illness

A clear and unmistakable warning that a bacterial infection is present is when previously clear nasal mucus turns a yellow or green color, or has a foul smell.

Bacterial infections frequently commence with largyngitis before spreading to bronchitis, ear infection, pneumonia, pharyngitis or strep throat, or tonsillitis. These complications frequently require medical treatment. Since they are primarily bacterial infections, they respond readily to antibiotics. Because complications may be either viral or bacterial, you should see a doctor without delay.

Other danger signs indicating a complication, and for which medical care should be sought, include these:

A fever over 101°F (38.3°C) with shaking, chills and coughing up of thick green, yellow or rust-colored, or foul-smelling phlegm.

A fever over 101°F (38.3°C) that lasts more than four days.

A persistent high fever over 102°F (38.8°C) with muscle aches that extends beyond three days.

A fever higher than 103°C (39.4°C).

Shortness of breath.

A sharp pain in the chest following a deep breath.

Coughing up of blood.

Severe cold symptoms or a sore throat which do not ameliorate after seven to eight days.

Throat pain in a child.

Breathing difficulty in a child with a cold, especially if accompanied by a hoarse cough.

A painful sore throat accompanied by:

—yellow-white pus spots on throat or tonsils.

—exposure to someone with strep throat.

—tender or swollen glands or bumps in front of the neck.

—a rash which appears during or after a sore throat.

—any past history of rheumatic heart disease, rheumatic fever, kidney disease or chronic lung disease such as emphysema or chronic bronchitis.

Appearance of any one or more of these warning signs may indicate a bacterial complication for which you should consult a physician without delay. You should also see a doctor if hoarseness from a cold has not improved after two weeks, especially if you smoke.

COMPLICATIONS THAT MAY FOLLOW A COLD OR INFLUENZA

Because the respiratory tract is a series of cavities (sinuses, lungs etc.), connected by air passages, viruses can spread from the nose to the sinuses and throat and into the middle ear trachea, larynx, bronchial tubes and lungs. Secondary infections spreading to these locations can cause complications, some quite serious.

Bronchitis

Bronchitis is inflammation of the mucous membranes that line the bronchial tubes, which carry air to the lungs. It is often caused by the common cold virus itself, in which case no medical cure is possible. However, a secondary bacterial infection is common. Symptoms often include a mild back or chest pain exacerbated by a deep, dry cough which brings up gray or yellow phlegm from the lungs. Bronchitis is also often accompanied by a fever which may last for as long as five days. Breathlessness and wheezing are other common symptoms.

Since bronchitis is not a lung infection, it is usually serious only if it becomes chronic. The usual treatment is to remain home in a warm room with humidified air and to bolster immunocompetence by practicing the same therapies recommended for a cold. If bronchitis does not begin to improve in forty-eight hours, or if you cough up blood, experience breathlessness or have a fever higher than 101°F, a physician should be consulted.

Lingering bronchitis symptoms often persist for two to three weeks after a cold or flu has ended.

Ear Infection

Each ear is connected to the throat by the Eustachian tube, a passage lined by mucosal tissue. During a cold or flu infection, the Eustachian tubes may become infected by bacteria. Due in part to their constant sniffling, ear infections are more common in children. A sharp pain in the ears caused by pressure build-up is the usual symptom.

Laryngitis

Laryngitis is a bacterial or viral infection of the larynx or voice box located at the top of the trachea (windpipe). The common cold virus is often the culprit, in which case medical treatment may be of little help. The infection causes inflammation of the mucous membranes of the larynx and vocal cords. Laryngitis is a common occurrence toward the end of a cold. Although fever and other flu-like symptoms may occur, the characteristic symptom is hoarseness which may be followed by loss of voice. When due to a viral infection, the voice returns as soon as the cold or flu ends. If voicelessness persists, a doctor should be consulted to determine the possible existence of a bacterial infection. Self-treatment includes staying at home and resting if possible, and bolstering immunocompetence by practicing the same therapies recommended for a cold.

Pneumonia

Pneumonia is an umbrella term used to describe a variety of forms of inflammation of the lungs, ranging from a mild complication following an upper respiratory tract infection to a life-threatening disease. In all cases, the alveoli or gas exchange cells lining the lungs become infected, either by a virus or bacteria. Bacterial pneumonia is fairly easy to cure with antibiotics, bed rest and soothing cough medicines but recovery from viral pneumonia can take weeks and may require breathing oxygen.

It is interesting to note that most cases of pneumonia occur in people with low immunocompetence.

Symptoms of pneumonia include a fever which may rise to 105°F with abrupt chills and sweating, a painful cough, a sharp chest pain while breathing, breathing difficulty while resting, blood in the sputum, and a bluish tinge to the skin.

Pneumonia is a common complication following a bout with cold or flu but in persons with low immunocompetence it can be precipitated by a variety of causes ranging from physical accident and trauma to emotional stress resulting from divorce or loss of a loved one.

Even in hospital, recovery can be speeded by bolstering immunocompetence through practicing Positivism and Deep Relaxation as described in Chapters 9 and 10.

Pharyngitis

This is inflammation of the pharynx, that portion of the throat above the larynx. Pharyngitis can be caused by either a virus or bacteria. Strep throat, a bacterial infection, is the most common and dangerous form of pharyngitis. Invariably, strep throat is accompanied by a high fever and an excruciatingly painful sore throat. Difficulty may be experienced in breathing, swallowing and speaking and the throat is red and raw. Although strep throat is not particularly common, it can lead to kidney disease, rheumatic heart disease or rheumatic fever. It can be positively diagnosed only by a two-day throat culture taken by a physician. Strep throat responds fairly readily to antibiotics.

Fortunately, most sore throats are not due to strep throat. Simply sore throat can be treated at home by resting the throat with a liquid diet, using slippery elm lozenges and gargling with salt water to relieve throat distress. You should also bolster immunocompetence by practicing Positivism and Deep Relaxation as described in Chapters 9 and 10. If symptoms persist longer than four to five days, consult a physician.

Sinusitis

Sinusitis is a common dysfunction which frequently occurs after a cold is complicated by a secondary bacterial infection. Sinusitis is inflammation of the mucous membranes of the air-filled sinus cavities, which are hollow spaces in the bones of the skull. The frontal sinuses are above the eyes, the maxillary sinuses behind the cheeks. They are lined by mucosal cells which produce mucus that drains into the throat.

When the nose is blocked by a cold, this discharge accumulates and blocks the nose still more. The sufferer must then breathe through the mouth and speech often becomes nasal. Tenderness and headache pain are also often experienced in the cheeks and forehead; below, behind and above the eyes; and in the upper teeth, especially in the rear upper jaw. Vision may also become blurred. Adding to the discomfort is further pain caused by irritated nerve endings in the sinuses themselves.

If the frontal sinuses are affected, headache pain usually appears over one or both eyes, especially upon waking or on bending forward. If the maxillary sinuses are affected, one or both cheeks may be tender and painful, and pain may be experienced in the upper jaw.

Sinusitis is not normally dangerous but when it appears together with a cold, and then continues to produce a copious green discharge after the cold ends, it may be due to a bacterial infection. Or it could be due to an allergy. If you suspect a bacterial infection, a physician can confirm sinusitis by X-ray diagnosis. Otherwise, treatment is similar to that for a cold.

Tonsillitis

Acute inflammation of the tonsils is usually caused by a bacteria although it is sometimes also due to a virus. Most doctors take a throat culture before prescribing antibiotics. Tonsillitis can usually be diagnosed by the red and inflamed condition of the tonsils and by swollen glands and tenderness under the neck and jaw. The condition is often accompanied by a feeling of being ill, by pain on swallowing and by an extremely sore throat, a headache, fever and chills.

Self-treatment includes resting at home in bed for one to two days, drinking plenty of liquids and bolstering immunocompetence with the same therapies recommended for a cold.

However, tonsillitis is primarily a disease of childhood, hence the treatment just described may not be possible. If symptoms persist longer than two days, consult a physician.

DYSFUNCTIONS WITH SYMPTOMS SIMILAR TO THOSE OF THE COMMON COLD

Several dysfunctions of the upper respiratory tract may be confused with cold or flu symptoms.

Allergic Rhinitis or Hayfever

When cold symptoms seem to persist for longer than fourteen days, the cause is more probably an allergy than a virus. Symptoms of allergic rhinitis include itchy, red, watery eyes which often swell; frequent sneezing; an itchy, runny nose; and a tickle in the back of the throat. The cause is hypersensitivity to an allergenic substance of which the most common are pollens, mold, animal danders, feathers, hair, household dust or chemicals, fungi, food preservatives and coloring, and such foods as beef, eggs, yeast, wheat, corn, chocolate, citrus or dairy products.

Allergic rhinitis may also be caused by prescription or OTC drugs.

The most common form of allergic rhinitis is hayfever, which is caused by pollen from trees and grass in spring, and ragweed in late summer and early fall.

Allergic rhinitis occurs when the immune system makes an exaggerated response to a foreign substance such as those just described. The immune system then responds to an allergen as though it were a disease-carrying invader. Histamine is released in the nasal passages which creates inflammation and congestion and excessive discharge of watery mucus from the fragile mucous membranes lining the nasal passages and sinuses. Simultaneously, B cells may begin to manufacture antibodies against the imaginary foe.

The entire immune system often mounts an attack

against the allergen comparable to that invoked by the common cold. Soon, the overzealous immune system is partially out of control. Billions of antibodies bind to the surface of mast cells in the nasal passageways. When allergens enter the nose, these cells explode, releasing more histamine to further amplify the rhinitis cycle.

Symptoms occur in the form of brief fifteen- to thirty-minute allergy attacks. Allergic rhinitis is most common at ages under forty and in persons having other allergy problems like asthma or eczema. It can be relieved by remaining indoors during the pollen season and by removing all sources of offending allergens from the house. Medical treatment is available but is not always successful. Since allergic rhinitis is caused by an exaggerated immune response, the one best way to end it permanently is to adopt the therapies for bolstering immunocompetence described in Chapters 7, 8, 9 and 10.

Asthma

Whereas hayfever is a reaction to an airborne allergen occurring in the eyes, nose and throat, asthma is a reaction to an airborne allergen occurring in the lungs and chest. Asthma can range from mild to life-threatening and is frequently precipitated by airborne pollen, seeds, pollutants or chemicals. It may also be triggered by emotional stress, infections and by vigorous outdoor exercise in cold weather. It is a common occupational disease among farmers, meat wrappers, bakers, cotton textile workers and others exposed to chemicals. Most of all, it is a disease of childhood and gradually disappears with advancing age.

The underlying cause of asthma is an exaggerated immune response to an airborne allergen and is identical to that just described under "Allergic Rhinitis."

The result is that when airways to the lungs are sensitive to an allergen, smooth muscles in the bronchial walls contract and constrict access of air to the lungs. Breathing difficulty results. Besides a tightness in the chest, and a shortness of breath, asthma symptoms often include a wheezing, unproductive cough. Attacks are sporadic and severity varies widely from one attack to the next. Severe attacks may cause breathing difficulties so intense that the lips turn blue, the pulse beats rapidly and the person sweats with anxiety.

Overall, asthma can range in severity from relatively mild cases which require no lifestyle restriction to life-endangering attacks which restrict many of the activities a person may engage in. Asthma often seems to run in families and sufferers are also often plagued by eczema or hayfever.

Although asthma is not medically curable, it can be relieved by OTC and prescription prophylactics, broncho-dilators or steroid drugs. Since these drugs are stronger than those used to treat colds or flu, both OTC and prescription drugs are best taken under the guidance of a physician.

Much can be done to permanently relieve asthma by staying indoors during the pollen season and by removing the source of other offending allergens such as animal danders, hairs, feathers and household dust. Since asthma is basically caused by an exaggerated immune response, the one best way to overcome it permanently is to adopt the therapies for bolstering immunocompetence described in Chapters 7, 8, 9 and 10.

OVERCOMING A COLD
OR FLU BY BOLSTERING
YOUR IMMUNOCOMPETENCE

If you have read this chapter so far, you will probably have concluded that the best way to shorten the duration of a cold or influenza, and to reduce the severity of its symptoms, is by enhancing one's immunocompetence.

This conclusion is perfectly correct. In case of a bacterial infection, a physician's antibiotics can replace a weak immune system. But so far, medical science can do nothing for a viral infection other than to soothe the discomfort of the symptoms. The fact is, that at this stage in scientific progress, we ourselves can do more to boost our immunocompetence than can any doctor or his drugs.

In recent years, a flood of new information has emerged from the leading edge of scientific research that links the immune system and our emotions to physical health. For instance, the new science of psychoneuroimmunology is actively exploring the relationships among the mind, body and immune system. Although no large-scale study has definitely established a mind-immunity link, the results of fifty or more small-scale studies all point, without a single exception, in the same direction. What they are essentially saying is that we can consciously choose to have a strong and powerful immune system by believing, thinking and behaving positively.

Confirming this conclusion are several carefully-controlled studies which have clearly demonstrated that depression and similar negative emotional states suppress the immune system. One study, for example, showed that moderately stressed or depressed women have 40 percent fewer virus-fighting killer T cells and 20 percent fewer helper T cells than normal. Although this book is concerned only with respiratory tract infections, the same stress mechanisms which can prolong a cold can also allow cancer and other infectious diseases to survive and proliferate. Thus whatever we do to overcome a cold or influenza, by bolstering immunocompetence will also significantly reduce our risk of getting cancer or other infectious disease.

The Mind—Body Connection

Other stress mechanisms triggered by beliefs, thoughts and emotional states can affect the central nervous system or the endocrine system, leading to vasomotor instability. When a person becomes enraged, angered or hostile, for example, the fight-or-flight response is invoked, causing constriction of arteries throughout the body. Within minutes, this condition can cut blood supplies to the heart muscle, precipitating sudden cardiac death, a heart attack or severe angina. The existence of this emotional link to heart disease has been thoroughly documented. But few researchers have bothered to investigate the fact that this same mechanism constricts blood vessels in nasal passages, reducing blood supply to the nose area and causing nasal congestion, and inhibiting the disease-resisting powers of nasal mucosa and of the cilia beating in nasal passages.

Gradually, piece by piece, the results of dozens of small scale studies are contributing to the total picture. We now know for example, that feeling lonely may also significantly suppress the immune system.

Other studies have demonstrated that positive beliefs, thoughts, emotions and attitudes can *enhance* immunocompetence. A number of studies have shown that antibody and helper T cell counts have been significantly boosted after subjects were given a few sessions of instruction in deep relaxation and creative mental imagery.

Basically, then, it has been found that prolonged stress, depression or other negative emotional states *suppress* the immune system while positive beliefs, thoughts, emotions and attitudes *enhance* our immunocompetence. While the benefits of Positivism have been most clearly identified in the link between emotions and immunity, strong and irrefutable evidence is also emerging to show that diet and exercise are also powerful tools for boosting immunity.

How Exercise Strengthens Immunity

Soon after beginning to exercise, for example, the adrenals secrete epinephrine, a hormone that stimulates immunity. Studies in athletic medicine have noted a clearly-defined relationship between vigorous physical exercise and an increase in resistance to infection. Several studies have clearly indicated that physically-active people have a significantly lower rate of cancer than sedentary people. It is speculated that exercise stimulates antibody production and also relaxes the arteries, allowing more blood to reach nasal passageways.

While the link between nutrition and stress is not quite as well defined, it has been shown that under stress, the body consumes key nutrients more rapidly than most diets can replace them. These deficiencies then inhibit replication of white cells and antibodies in the vast numbers required to launch a counterattack against invading infections.

For example, vitamin C increases interferon in the blood stream, and is believed to stimulate interferon production by infected cells. Vitamins A and E, and the entire B-complex, all provide essential nutritional support to a beleaguered immune system as do such key minerals as calcium, magnesium, iron and zinc.

The long duration of Bob Rhinehart's cold, described blow-by-blow earlier, was due to Bob's poor immunocompetence. Besides holding many negative beliefs and experiencing frequent negative emotions, Bob was completely indifferent to the need for exercise and his diet was largely based on high-risk and junk foods.

Even though colds and flu are confined to the respiratory tract, they set off an immune response that affects not only the entire body but the Whole Person. The way we respond to events in our lives, and the extent to which we exercise and the way we eat, have more to do with shortening the duration of a cold or flu than any therapy which focuses only on the infected area.

In fact, whatever we do to enhance the fitness and health of either body or mind fortifies the immune system also. The immune system exactly mirrors the health of our body-mind continuum. When we feed and care for our bodies, and when we seek peace and contentment instead of emotional turmoil, our immunocompetence attains its optimal peak.

Colds Are a Whole Person Dysfunction

As a result, the only successful way to overcome a cold or flu in a minimum of time is to use a Whole Person approach. Known also as holistic healing, this means that we ourselves must intervene on the emotional, physical and nutritional levels simultaneously.

After absorbing this chapter, you should now be familiar with the entire disease process of upper respiratory tract viral infections. This know-how can give you a tremendous feeling of power over any case of cold or flu you may catch. You can easily recognize the few danger signals that may indicate a medical emergency. You should also be able to confidently handle your own home treatment. And you can speed up recovery by using natural, alternative-healing techniques based on mental, physical and emotional approaches. All of these healing therapies are things we can easily do for ourselves at nominal cost.

Chapter by chapter, the remainder of this book describes the Whole Person approach to shortening the duration of a cold or flu and to minimizing and soothing the severity of the symptoms. Using this methodology, you can avoid most of the misery and discomfort and, in the case of a cold, continue to go to work with undiminished energy. Included in the chapters which follow are dozens of natural, do-it-yourself remedies for soothing away the pain and discomfort of cold and flu symptoms. Most of these are less dangerous and more successful than the majority of commercial cough and cold remedies. Everything you need to know to successfully treat an upper respiratory tract infection at home is described within these pages.

Since medical care is an integral part of the holistic approach to healing, the next chapter discusses the pros and cons of prescription and OTC cough and cold remedies.

4 The Medical Approach

A century ago, physicians used to say that, "untreated, a cold is usually over in a week, treated it should last seven days."

Most doctors are still giving the same advice. Despite giant strides in curing other types of viral infections, as this was written, medical science could do little more than ease the distress of cold and flu symptoms. No cure has been discovered nor had any drug been found to shorten the duration of a cold or influenza.

Moreover, almost every medication developed to alleviate cold or flu symptoms has some degree of adverse side effects. For example, if use is prolonged, almost every medication for any type of upper respiratory tract dysfunction will eventually aggravate the very symptoms it is designed to relieve. And a review panel appointed by the FDA has found hundreds of OTC remedies for respiratory infections to be both unsafe and ineffective.

Several authorities have suggested that most, if not all,

remedies for colds, coughs, flu, asthma, hayfever and other respiratory dysfunctions are immuno-suppressants. Since this applies to both OTC and prescription medications, it suggests that most drugs (excluding only antibiotics) actually prolong an infection and intensify the overall symptoms.

Medicine's most significant contribution has been in preventing respiratory infections through vaccines, sprays and other medications.

The Interferon Spray

The newest contribution to cold prevention is the interferon nasal spray developed simultaneously at the University of Virginia and the University of Adelaide, Australia. The two universities tested a total of 150 families, each composed of four or more people living in a household setting. Whenever a household member came down with cold symptoms, the others sprayed their nasal passages with alpha-interferon for a period of seven days.

Interferon (described in Chapter 3) is released by nasal cells infected by viruses to immunize nearby cells from viral attack. Results of the spray have been encouraging. The studies showed that interferon reduced incidence of rhinovirus colds by 80 percent. Over the six to eight months test period, interferon-protected families had 40 percent fewer colds than comparable control-group families.

But the interferon spray will not cure a cold once symptoms appear. During tests, users experienced irritation and minor nasal bleeding some 10 percent of the time, especially when using the spray for more than seven days. The spray may not be feasible for children. Since colds are contagious before symptoms appear, the spray may not protect during this period. Although interferon is being produced by genetic engineering, its cost may still be fairly high. FDA approval could be delayed and if the spray is available by prescription only, it could be financially out of reach of many people. The spray appears usable only for seven days at a time after which the user is exposed to risk of catching cold again until the effects of the spray wear off and it can be used for another seven-day period. Finally, even when used, it protects against only 40 percent of the overall risk of catching cold.

The interferon spray is of no help in alleviating cold symptoms, though it might possibly shorten the duration of a cold by reducing the number of cells a virus can infect.

Monoclonal Antibodies

Another possible way to prevent the common cold is based on the discovery that 90 percent of rhinoviruses bind to one type of receptor in nasal cells. It is also known that monoclonal antibodies will also bind to this same receptor. Several scientists have speculated that if enough monoclonal antibodies are released into the nose, they will block all receptors and prevent access to the viruses.

To test this theory, a group of volunteers took nose drops containing monoclonal antibodies ten times over a thirty-nine-hour period. A control group took nothing. Both groups were then exposed to a rhinovirus.

Only nine of the thirteen-member test group caught colds compared to eleven of the thirteen-member control group. However, the test group did have significantly milder symptoms. While the study suggests that monoclonal antibodies can indeed block cell receptors, results as yet do not justify their use as a cold prophylactic.

Drug WIN 51,711

Drug WIN 51,711, developed by a leading pharmaceutical manufacturer, has demonstrated broad antiviral effects against the rhinovirus as well as against a wide spectrum of related viral infections. An analog of the drug binds to a site on the surface of the rhinovirus, preventing it from shedding its protein coat and, as a result, from being able to replicate.

Although this may sound promising, by the time the drug is taken and becomes effective, the worst of a cold may be over.

The eventual outcome may be that both the interferon spray and WIN 51,711 will be combined with related antiviral compounds to provide a shotgun approach to preventing and curing the common cold. Meanwhile, it seems fairly safe to assume that a medical cure for the common cold or flu still lies in the distant, unforeseeable future.

A GUIDE TO VACCINES FOR RESPIRATORY DISEASES

Vaccines have been developed against influenza, pneumonia and some allergies. Thus far, efforts to produce a cold vaccine have been unsuccessful although scientists claim to have identified a relatively stable part of the cold virus's outer coat against which a vaccine may one day be developed.

Influenza Vaccine

By identifying the types and variants of influenza virus, scientists have developed an effective vaccine. But since the virus changes its antigen every year, immunity seldom lasts for more than twelve months. At present, the vaccine is also effective against only a single variant of the disease (a statement subject to future change).

Since influenza vaccine must be produced months in advance, and no one knows exactly which variant will predominate next winter, predicting which vaccine to manufacture is an inexact science. The U.S. Centers for Disease Control (CDC) continually monitor new flu mutations throughout the world. Each spring, CDC respresentatives meet with influenza advisory committees to try to determine which strain of virus to include in next season's vaccine.

Despite this pooling of experience, they can still be wide of the mark. When the swine flu appeared in 1976 its genetic make-up closely resembled that of the Spanish flu that caused the worldwide epidemic of 1918. The U.S. Government prepared to vaccinate all Americans against what seemed like a particularly virulent rogue virus. But it all turned out to be a false alarm and some people who received the vaccine experienced neurological problems.

Nor is flu vaccine entirely free of side effects. Between four and twelve percent of recipients have experienced mild flu symptoms for twenty four hours after injections. More rarely, people who are sensitive to eggs may develop a serious allergic reaction. Many people also experience pain and tenderness at the inoculation site.

Most vaccine in use today is bivalent, implying that it is effective against a variant of either A or B types. However, significant protection seldom lasts longer than six months and a person is still only immune to the mainstream variant. Inoculation provides little immunity should a new subtype appear. And some researchers believe that vaccines tend only to serve to help promote evolution of new flu virus strains.

If you do decide to be vaccinated against flu, remember that it takes some fourteen days for the immune system to produce antibodies in response to the injection. For maximum protection, you should be vaccinated by mid-October.

The prescription drug Amatadine is also used to prevent Type A influenza in high risk populations. It can be taken up to two days after symptoms appear. However, Amatadine may cause side effects ranging from poor concentration to mild headaches, insomnia or irritability.

Pneumonia Vaccine

A vaccine was developed in 1983 which has proved effective against 87.5 percent of bacterial pneumonia. It is recommended for the elderly and other high risk persons. Once given, the inoculation is effective for a period of five years. Side effects have included arm soreness while a small number of recipients have experienced short term, low-grade fever.

Allergy Shots

Shots are available to reduce sensitivity to severe allergic rhinitis. The procedure first requires an allergist or physician to identify the offending allergen by skin or other test. A small amount of the allergenic substance is then injected into the bloodstream, causing the immune system to form blocking antibodies. These antibodies reduce any subsequent immune response to the allergenic substance.

However, the testing and inoculation process is expensive and time-consuming while the FDA review panel found that many allergenic extracts used for injections were ineffective.

Steroid Drugs

Prescribed for relief of some cases of allergic rhinitis and asthma, steroid drugs have been found to directly suppress the immune system.

Take Two Aspirin and Drink Plenty of Fluids

Meanwhile, the standard medical treatment for either a cold or flu is to drink plenty of fluids, to take an aspirin every four hours, and—if fever is present—to stay in bed. (Usually, fever occurs only with flu.)

Aspirin apart, this is sound advice. Drink plenty of water or fresh vegetable or diluted fruit juices. If you have a fever, stay in bed until your temperature drops to normal. And although the benefits of aspirin are debatable, taking one every four hours can temporarily relieve the discomfort of muscular aches and pains and it may lower your fever.

However, aspirin has such toxicity that if it were discovered today, many authorities believe it would be available only by prescription. Aspirin relieves pain by blocking production of prostaglandins, hormone-like substances released by the body to produce inflammation. Aspirin, or its substitute acetaminophen, are both used to temporarily relieve muscle ache, fever and chills, throat distress and fatigue.

Unless you are allergic to aspirin, you will probably find it effective. But in suppressing symptoms such as fever or inflammation, aspirin may well be counter-productive to the body's efforts to heal itself. For example, reducing fever may prolong the infection. Likewise, by suppressing prostaglandin production throughout the body, aspirin may inhibit the supply of prostaglandins that protect the stomach lining, thereby causing stomach upset and possible mild bleeding.

The continued use of aspirin to relieve cold or flu may lead to reduced immunocompetence.

For example, nasal inflammation is an essential defense mechanism of the immune system and is used to limit spread of infection. In the process, sensory nerves are compressed by the swelling and pain results. Aspirin relieves the swelling by destroying a key enzyme required for the synthesis of the prostaglandin that causes inflammation. By preventing inflammation, aspirin relieves pressure on nerves and pain disappears. In the process, aspirin retards the healing of viral infections. In fact, continuous aspirin use exacerbates immunodeficiency and it reduces immunocompetence.

If aspirin is held in the mouth instead of being swallowed immediately, it can cause burning and irritation to the lining of the mouth and throat. It can also cause ringing in the ears and irritation to ulcers. Aspirin substitutes have also caused a drop in blood pressure with possible damage to liver or kidneys.

Youngsters below the early twenties in age are also being urged to avoid taking aspirin or salicylate-containing medication when suffering from flu-like symptoms as the drug has been linked with Reye's Syndrome, a dangerous neurological disease that can cause death or lifelong impairment of the liver or brain.

Some researchers also suspect that aspirin causes an increase in the number of viruses in the nose. While a small amount over a short period can probably be tolerated without serious harm, aspirin or its substitutes do nothing at all to cure or shorten the duration of a cold or influenza.

Small doses of codeine will also provide temporary relief from cough symptoms and the aches and pains of flu. But codeine has considerable toxicity and is available as a single ingredient drug only by prescription.

Many OTC Remedies Found Worthless

In recent years, a panel of experts appointed by the FDA has reviewed the effectiveness, safety and accuracy of claims made on the labels of all OTC remedies for cough, colds and other respiratory ailments. Literally hundreds of specific products were found unsafe and ineffective and have been removed from the market. About those remaining on drugstore and pharmacy shelves, the FDA has released the following advice.

Medications consisting of a single ingredient tend to be more effective than those which attempt a shotgun approach by claiming to have "a combination of medically-active ingredients." Many of the ingredients are often inappropriate for relief of cold symptoms. A brew of different drugs may also interact and work against each other, or cancel out each other's benefits. They may also compound side effects. For example, large concentrations of caffeine are often included to offset the drowsiness produced by antihistamines which, in turn, offer no benefit at all to cold sufferers and are effective only against allergies. Many cold remedies contain a mix of antihistamine, pain relievers and nasal decongestants, usually in amounts too small to be effective.

If you do decide to use an OTC preparation, aim for a single-ingredient product designed specifically for the symptom you wish to relieve. Avoid a mix of many drugs, the only aim of which is to support the extravagant advertising claim on the product's label.

Be aware, also, that many OTC nose and throat preparations may irritate the mucous membranes and prolong infection. Among the most common side effects of OTC cold, cough and hayfever remedies are drowsiness, dry mouth, headaches, nausea, irregular heartbeat, blurred vision, skin rash, increased nervousness, mood alterations and raised blood pressure. To offset these side effects, some preparations contain aspirin substitutes.

To help you evaluate each type of cold medication, here is a rundown on their pros and cons. They are taken from FDA reports, the *Physician's Desk Reference* and other dependable medical sources.

Anticholinergenics

Often using drugs like belladonna alkaloids or atropine sulphate, these cold remedies dry up watery secretions in the eyes and nose. In doing so, they may cause dried-up plugs of nasal secretions to block air passages or to cause coughing. Side effects have included blurred vision, rapid heartbeat, confusion, insomnia, constipation, and dry mouth. The FDA panel considered these unsuitable for people with asthma, glaucoma or bladder problems.

Antitussives (Cough Suppressants)

Towards the end of a cold, a barking, nonproductive cough may appear that disturbs sleep. It can be controlled by the narcotic-free suppressant dextromethorphan or by the prescription drug codeine, both of which suppress the cough center in the brain. These medications should not be used for chronic coughs caused by asthma, emphysema or smoking. Codeine is also a narcotic that may produce drowsiness, vomiting, nausea, constipation and light-headedness.

Decongestants

Nasal decongestants in the form of sprays, nose drops or tablets shrink and dry out swollen mucous membranes in the nose and sinuses and liquify dried-up mucus.

OTC decongestants come in two varieties: those containing antihistamine which are recommended for allergy and hayfever relief; and those which do not employ antihistamine and are recommended for relief of cold symptoms. Since antihistamine does nothing for cold relief, you should avoid using a decongestant containing antihistamine to relieve a stuffed-up nose due to a cold. It's important to realize that cold-relief decongestants perform only a single function: by constricting large blood vessels in nasal passages, they cause the airways to open up. Thus decongestants will only relieve a stuffy nose. In practice, they are worth using only if the nose is so badly stuffed up that breathing is difficult or sleep is interfered with (or possibly when the ears are affected). The majority have such a variety of side effects that many doctors recommend that you keep blowing the nose gently rather than use a decongestant.

Most OTC nose sprays make you feel better for a short while. But the effects soon wear off, leaving you feeling worse than before. This shortcoming frequently leads to overuse of sprays which can damage nasal membranes. Worse still, prolonged use dilates the blood vessels, creating a condition of rebound congestion and possible dependency. Hence, most doctors warn that you should not use a nasal decongestant for more than three days at a time. Otherwise, prolonged use can lead to overproduction of mucus and to scar tissue in nasal passages.

Some nose drops and nasal sprays also irritate mucosa lining nose and throat passages, changing the pH balance from acidic to alkaline, which can enhance risk of a bacterial infection. Some people who take nosedrops for more than three days often experience a rebound effect in which the nasal mucosa swells even more. Prolonged use of nose drops may lead to permanently swollen mucous membranes.

Among side effects attributed to decongestants are the stimulation of the heart and pulse rates and the feeling of being "high." Decongestants recommended for allergy relief have caused skipped heart beat, insomnia and nervousness. Many decongestants are not suitable for those with hypertension, irregular heartbeat, glaucoma or difficulty in urinating.

Since only antihistamine is effective against hayfever and allergies, these conditions should not be treated with topical decongestants such as inhalers, sprays or nose drops which contain ingredients designed to relieve cold symptoms. Thus decongestants recommended for allergy relief are usually ineffective for a cold. Never share a nasal spray or inhaler with anyone else as it can transfer cold and flu viruses.

Oral decongestants are primarily used to relieve ear fullness or muffled hearing as well as swollen nasal, throat and sinus tissues. To be really effective, however, the dosage must be so high that it makes a person feel hyper and all wired-up. Oral decongestants may also cause insomnia. The relatively high dosage of drugs used in oral decongestants may also increase blood pressure significantly. As a result, oral decongestants are not recommended for those with heart disease, hypertension, diabetes or thyroid disorders. Oral formulas may also interfere with some antihypertensive prescription drugs which can become addictive.

In view of these risks, most doctors consider that nasal sprays, inhalants and nose drops are safer and more effective when used solely for relieving a badly stuffed-up nose.

Expectorants

Expectorants raise secretions from the bronchial airways so that they can be expectorated. Cough mixtures containing Guaifenesin are considered fairly effective.

Mouthwashes and Gargles

Mouthwashes and gargles will briefly freshen the mouth and throat but the benefit is mostly cosmetic. However, some brands provide temporary pain relief.

Throat Lozenges and Sprays

Lozenges can keep the throat moist but so can chewing hard candy. Throat sprays, or lozenges containing pain relievers, can provide temporary relief for the distress of a sore throat. But lozenges containing a mix of pain relievers, decongestants and cough suppressants are seldom effective as the ingredients often nullify each other.

Because sprays and lozenges containing pain relievers may mask a serious throat infection such as strep throat, you are advised to limit their use to a maximum of forty-eight hours.

Children should never be given the full adult dosage of any OTC medication. Children aged six to eleven require only half the adult dose while those two to five may be given one-fourth the recommended adult dose. Infants under two should be given medication only on a physician's advice.

Similar caveats apply to almost all OTC medications for dysfunctions with symptoms that may be confused with those of the common cold.

Antihistamines

Antihistamines reduce swollen membranes, congestion, running nose, sneezing, postnasal drip and itchy, watery eyes *due to allergic rhinitis* by blocking the effects of prostaglandins produced by histamine. Antihistamines are available in tablets, capsules or liquid OTC remedies and may be included in anti-sneezing preparations. While anti-histamines are effective in relieving hayfever and similar types of allergic rhinitis, they are most effective in single-ingredient medications that contain only antihistamine. Multi-ingredient products can compound side effects while ingredients other than antihistamine have no benefits for allergic rhinitis.

The most common side effect of antihistamines is drowsiness. Some antihistamines, in fact, are used to induce sleep. Worth knowing is that products using brom-pheniramine maleate or chlorpheniramine maleate seem to cause least drowsiness. Less common side effects include low blood pressure, headaches, loss of coordination, nausea, dizziness, blurred vision, constriction of small blood vessels, anxiety, loss of appetite and dryness of nose, throat and mouth. This dryness may extend to bronchial tissue, making it difficult to raise mucus from the chest without severe coughing.

Since antihistamines dry up secretions which may block airways and increase breathing difficulties, antihista-mines should not be used by those with asthma. Nor should antihistamines be used by anyone with glaucoma or an enlarged prostate unless prescribed by a physician; and antihistamines may cause nervousness, restlessness and insomnia in children.

Although antihistamines prevent the discomfort of hayfever, in doing so they may retard the healing process.

Antihistamines used in anti-sneezing preparations may, in the process of inhibiting sneezing, actually thicken mucus and worsen cold symptoms. OTC cold remedies which include antihistamines also carry an unsuspected hazard: they may suppress certain cold or flu symptoms, giving the impression that one has recovered. A person may then decide to get up and return to work, which could increase the risk of complications.

Asthma Medications

Both OTC and prescription drugs for asthma are stronger than those used for colds or flu and should be taken only under the guidance of a physician. The prescription drug Theophylline is widely used but it has a critically narrow dosage range; too little has no effect while too much causes a wide range of serious side effects ranging from irregular heartbeat to vomiting, stomach pains, jitters, insomnia, headaches or even seizures.

Ephedrine, used in most OTC asthma remedies, is considered less effective. To offset its stimulating effects, phenobarbital, a powerful sedative, is often added. The combination may affect the heart and nervous system, producing tremor, insomnia and loss of appetite.

These and similar drugs used for asthma are known as bronchodilators for their action in relaxing the smooth muscles of lung air passages, causing them to dilate and make breathing easier. They will not relieve hayfever. As always, single ingredient OTC products are most effective.

Bronchodilators are availale in tablet or elixir form, or as inhalers. Most OTC inhalant bronchodilators contain epinephrine, which has numerous side effects and to which the airways soon develop a tolerance. Because bronchodilators can affect the heart and nervous system, they may not be suitable for those with hypertension, heart disease, thyroid disease, diabetes and glaucoma, or for men with an enlarged prostate.

Grim Effects of Medicines

From all this we may conclude that every drug is a two-edged sword which may offset possible benefits by adverse side effects. Because no drug can cure or shorten the duration of a cold or flu, the temporary benefits drugs may afford frequently do *not* outweigh the potential harm they may cause.

The fact that many doctors themselves recommend avoiding OTC or prescription medications for simple colds or flu is sufficient testimony that the medical approach to overcoming these infections has little to offer the average victim. Only in case of danger signals, an emergency or a complication can a doctor really be of help.

Furthermore, the function of many OTC cold remedies can be duplicated—without risk of side effects or suppression of the immune system—by natural therapies described in the remainder of this book. Herbal remedies, described in Chapter 6, are especially helpful in relieving symptoms without the side effects and the potential immunosuppression of drugs.

5 The Nutritional Approach

Supportive nutrition is essential if the immune system is to end viral infection swiftly. A number of small-scale studies all appear to confirm that vitamin and mineral deficiencies are partly responsible for suppression of the immune system which prolongs the severity and duration of colds and flu.

Other studies are showing that whenever the body is stressed by an infection, key nutrients such as vitamins A and C, and the mineral zinc, may be depleted more rapidly than the average diet can replenish them. This deficiency then further lowers immunocompetence. Although results are preliminary, these studies are consistent with the existence of a public health problem of deficiency in nutrients that support immunocompetence.

Unless at least 80 percent of your diet consists of fresh fruits, vegetables, nuts, seeds, whole grains and legumes, your body may be unable to absorb sufficient essential nutrients from the food you eat. Recent surveys have shown that a high intake of polyunsaturated fat, in the form of pressed vegetable oils, can be immunosuppressive while the Standard American Diet with its emphasis on meat fats, dairy foods, eggs, fried foods and other animal products tends to be deficient in such key nutrients as vitamins A and C and zinc. Each of these appears essential to a high level of immunocompetence. Even if your diet were nutritionally adequate, such influences as sugar, saturated fats, alcohol, caffeine, The Pill, diuretics and other medications or stimulants can inhibit absorption of key nutrients.

For those unable or unwilling to upgrade their diet as described in Chapter 9, nutritional supplements offer an alternative way to improve immunocompetence.

Nutrients That Build Immunocompetence

For example, in a French study of 100 healthy people aged over sixty, doctors found that the higher the vitamin A content in the bloodstream, the greater was the body's ability to produce helper T cells. Subjects with the highest vitamin A content in blood plasma had the highest immunocompetence. The same researchers confirmed that the higher a person's concentration of vitamin E in the blood plasma, the fewer the number of infections that person had experienced in the preceding three years.

Several studies on lab animals have confirmed that in animals deprived of vitamin A, the immune system is suppressed while supplementation with vitamin A bolstered immunocompetence in the test animals.

Other studies have demonstrated that a subtle zinc deficiency underlies a variety of impaired immunoresponse functions, and that fewer than fifty per cent of Americans have an adequate intake of dietary zinc.

Part of the controversy concerning claims that vitamin C will subdue cold symptoms arises from the difficulty in using lab animals for vitamin C testing. Unlike humans, most lab animals synthesize copious amounts of vitamin C in their bodies, making it impossible to measure the results of supplementation.

It is because humans are believed to have lost the ability to synthesize vitamin C due to a mutation during evolution that the need for vitamin C supplementation has become apparent.

In support of this concept, numerous tests on humans have confirmed that people who maintain higher levels of vitamin C in their bodies experience fewer respiratory infections; and if they do catch a cold, symptoms tend to be twenty to thirty percent less severe.

For example, a study made by the Naval Medical Research Institute, Bethesda, Maryland, and reported in the *Journal of Applied Nutrition* (vol. 34, no 1, 1982) tested the plasma vitamin C levels of twenty-eight men on a submarine during a sixty-eight-day patrol. Among those with the lowest vitamin C levels, twice as many experienced common cold symptoms as among those with the highest vitamin C levels.

Another study made in Australia, and reported in the *Medical Journal of Australia* (Oct 17, 1981) revealed that when cold sufferers were given one gram of vitamin C per day, the duration of their infection was reduced by 19 percent.

Even more convincing results were obtained in a large, carefully-controlled study made by Dr. Terence W. Anderson of the University of Toronto School of Hygiene in 1971–1972. After observing results of over 4,000 subjects in a series of three tests, each employing varying amounts of vitamin C, the overall conclusion was that regardless of the amount of vitamin C taken, the cold symptoms of those taking the vitamin were reduced by 30 percent.

Cold-Fighting Nutrients

The consensus of many similar studies is that vitamin C stimulates production of interferon; that it enhances the ability of the thymus gland to produce T cells; that it helps detoxify surplus histamine; and that it bolsters bacterial phagocytosis (ability of phagocytes to destroy bacteria). Doses of 2 to 3 grams have produced significant increases in immunocompetence.

As a result, vitamin C has become the best known dietary factor affecting immunity. On coming down with a cold, many people are now taking C instead of aspirin. Which is understandable when you consider that several carefully-conducted medical studies have shown that a mild viral infection, such as a smallpox inoculation, causes a significant depletion in vitamins A and C in the bloodstream.

While the results of studies like those just quoted have confirmed the benefits of vitamins A and C, and of zinc in treating colds, the lack of any large-scale scientifically endorsed proof seems due more to the nature of the scientific method than to any doubt about the nutrient's effectiveness. Any study is limited to testing only a single variable. Thus only a single vitamin or mineral can be tested at a time. By contrast, vitamins and minerals interact biologically, and work synergistically with each other, to produce results far greater than that of any single nutrient acting alone. Taken together, vitamins A, C, E and the B-complex plus zinc and other key minerals, appear to complement the other to produce overall results far in excess of any single nutrient studies so far recorded.

Super Nutrition for Cold Therapy

To really bolster our immunocompetence, we need a sufficiency of the following nutrients. (The recommended daily amounts given below are for adults while treating a cold. Lesser amounts may be sufficient for daily maintenance.)

Vitamin A	10,000 IU
B-complex vitamins including B1, B6, pantothenic acid, B12, folate and PABA.	as suggested
Vitamin C	as suggested
Vitamin D	400 IU
Vitamin E	200 IU
Calcium	1,000 mg
Iron	25 mg
Magnesium	500 mg
Selenium	100 mcg
Zinc	as suggested

While reduced immunocompetence has been clearly linked with a deficiency of vitamins A and C and with zinc, adequate amounts of the entire spectrum of nutrients listed above is recommended by many nutritionists to ensure complete nutritional support in reducing the severity and duration of cold symptoms.

To enable you to maximize their properties, here is a brief rundown of the most important nutrients known to enhance immunocompetence.

Vitamin A

Vitamin A plays a key role in maintaining the integrity of epithelial cells lining the mucosal tissues of respiratory passages. A deficiency of A causes these cells to dry out and become increasingly susceptible to viral penetration.

Vitamin A is also essential for optimal functioning of the adrenal, thyroid and thymus glands, each vital to immunocompetence. Vitamin A stimulates the thymus to produce more T cells. A healthy thyroid gland is essential for converting beta-carotene in food into additional vitamin A for use by the body. And without an adequate supply of vitamin A, the adrenal glands may secrete cortisol which directly suppresses the immune system.

While the RDA for vitamin A is 5,000 IU daily, or 8,000 IU for pregnant women, many nutritionists believe that an intake of 10 to 15,000 IU would be more appropriate during a cold.

Vitamin B Complex

A deficiency of B-complex components, especially B1, B5, B6, B12, folic acid and PABA, have been clearly linked to impairment of the immune system in many animal species. Particularly when B1, B5 and B6 are low in the bloodstream, immunocompetence has been found to fall off. A lack of vitamin B1 (thiamine) can also cause mild depression which has a detrimental effect on immunity. Vitamin B5 (pantothenic acid) has helped relieve many severe cases of hayfever; for this purpose, you should begin taking it one month before the hayfever season begins. And PABA is a B-complex component which acts as an anti-inflammatory agent.

It is not necessary to take large amounts of any single B vitamin. However, when intake of any single B vitamin is increased, the entire spectrum of the B complex should be increased proportionately. Hence B-vitamins are best taken in the form of a timed-release B-complex supplement containing the entire range of B-components.

Vitamin C

In 1970, Nobel Laureate Linus Pauling started a medical controversy with his book *Vitamin C and the Common Cold*. Few people today question that vitamin C relieves symptoms and shortens the duration of the common cold. But both the public and the scientific community are concerned by the ever-increasing dosages being recommended by many contemporary practitioners.

For example, at first Pauling recommended 250 to 1,000 mg of ascorbic acid (vitamin C) daily to prevent colds and infections. Should a cold appear, he recommended increasing intake to 1 to 10 g daily, depending on one's personal tolerance to vitamin C and on the severity of the infection. Nowadays, Pauling recommends 10 g a day as a prophylactic dose, while if you get a cold, the dose is 2 g per hour.

Meanwhile, other doctors have suggested amounts as high as 25 to 100 g per day to be taken during a cold. Some doctors find that 80 to 90 percent of the amount you can tolerate without getting diarrhea is effective.

During controlled trials, these enormous doses have shown little discernible advantage over smaller amounts.

As a result, many nutritionists today believe that, in their zeal to prove its cold-fighting properties, the pioneers of vitamin C therapy have overlooked two important factors. They are:

1. When tested under controlled conditions, relatively small daily doses of vitamin C (in the 3 to 5 g range) have achieved the same results as megadoses. Moreover, these very large doses may cause stomach gas, heartburn or diarrhea.

2. To achieve its maximum biological activity, vitamin C must interact with adequate amounts of other vitamins and minerals such as vitamin A and E, the B-complex and zinc. By focusing exclusively on vitamin

C, and ignoring the role of these other essential nutrients, vitamin C therapists are failing to maximize the full benefits of vitamin C. By working synergistically with other essential nutrients, smaller amounts of vitamin C can enhance immunocompetence more effectively than can large doses of vitamin C alone.

Assuming that a cold sufferer has a satisfactory intake of all other essential nutrients—especially vitamins A and E, the B-complex and zinc—what is the optimal amount of vitamin C to take? Let us begin by defining this as "holistic vitamin C therapy," implying a therapy in which all other vitamins and minerals play a supportive role in the healing properties of vitamin C.

Based on this concept, many nutritionists today are recommending that, as a prophylactic measure during the cold season, 250 mg should be taken with each major meal, or a total of three 250 mg tablets per day. (Two hundred and fifty milligram amounts can be made by slicing a 500 mg tablet in half.)

On the first appearance of cold symptoms, the consensus is to begin by taking one gram of vitamin C. After that, continue taking 500 mg every two-and-a-half hours throughout the time you are awake. On retiring, take a one gram (1,000 mg) timed-release capsule of vitamin C. If you wake in the middle of the night, take another. Resume the 500 mg per two-and-a-half-hour-routine immediately on waking in the morning.

If timed-release one-gram capsules are not available, take an extra 500 mg tablet on retiring provided you have not taken any vitamin C dosage within the previous hour. If you wake in the middle of the night, take another. If you do not wake during the night, take 750 mg of vitamin C on rising, then resume the 500 mg every two-and-a-half hour-routine.

For vitamin C to be effective, you must maintain a

surplus in the bloodstream at all times. Because the kidneys strain out all superfluous vitamin C from the bloodstream in about three hours, many nutritionists recommend replenishing the supply every two-and-a-half to three hours. In this way, you can maintain an above-average vitamin C level in your bloodstream throughout most of the twenty-four hours.

If you have *not* been taking the 750 mg daily prophylactic dose of vitamin C, and should a cold appear, start off by taking one gram of vitamin C. Two and a half hours later, take another one gram dose. Then continue taking 500 mg every two-and-a-half hours as in the program just described.

Whether or not you have been taking the 750 mg prophylactic dose, the important thing is to commence the 500 mg per two-and-a-half-hour routine as swiftly as possible after the first recognizable cold symptom appears.

Based on observations of subjects who have commenced holistic vitamin C therapy within an hour of the appearance of cold symptoms, after only eighteen hours of therapy at least 80 percent of the usual cold symptoms had failed to materialize.

After thirty-six hours of holistic vitamin C therapy, almost all cold symptoms should have disappeared.

Assuming that cold symptoms *have* largely disappeared, on the fourth and fifth days take one 500 mg tablet of vitamin C every three hours. Continue taking a one-gram timed-release capsule of vitamin C at bedtime; alternatively, if you have not taken a dose of vitamin C in the previous one-and-a-half-hours, you can take an extra 500 mg tablet. Even if you do not wake during the night, take only a 500 mg tablet in the morning.

Most people who follow holistic vitamin C therapy, and who take the other essential nutrients listed earlier in this chapter, find they are free of all cold symptoms by the third day.

However, if cold symptoms do not disappear, continue taking 500 mg of vitamin C every three hours.

Starting either on the fifth day, or when cold symptoms have disappeared, continue to take 400 mg of vitamin C every three hours. (You can make a 400 mg dosage by slicing one fifth off a 500 mg tablet.) Continue this dosage through the end of the sixth day. You can still take a one-gram timed-release capsule at bedtime; or in lieu of that an extra 400 mg tablet, provided over two hours has elapsed since you last took vitamin C. Starting on the seventh day, take 250 mg of vitamin C every three hours. You can still take a one-gram timed-release capsule at bedtime; or in lieu of it, a 250 mg tablet provided over two hours has elapsed since last taking vitamin C.

On the twelfth day, you can resume your regular prophylactic dose of 250 mg three times a day.

To achieve results, holistic vitamin C therapy must be started within twenty-four hours of the first appearance of cold symptoms. If more than twenty-four hours have elapsed, holistic vitamin C therapy will probably be only fifty percent effective. If forty-eight hours have elapsed, it's too late.

The idea is to maintain a constant level of vitamin C in the bloodstream. When cold symptoms have disappeared, you can begin to taper off the dosage until by the twelfth day, you are back to your prophylactic dosage of 250 mg three times a day.

The effectiveness of these smaller amounts of vitamin C is based on the assumption that you will take the other suggested essential nutrients in the amounts suggested. A good way to take them is in the form of a multiple vitamin-mineral supplement which should be taken daily throughout the cold season. However, you will require a separate full spectrum B-complex timed-release capsule. Once a cold begins, zinc should be taken in the form of zinc gluconate lozenges as described later. During a cold, do be sure you are getting at least 10,000 IU of vitamin A each day. If you have any doubts, eat a large raw carrot each day.

Some physicians have advised that you should not eat over half a pint of yogurt or buttermilk during the eight hours prior to starting vitamin C cold treatment. Others have suggested that people with an ulcer, or other digestive tract disease or problems, should employ vitamin C therapy only under a physician's guidance.

Linus Pauling and others recommended using plain abscorbic acid, the cheapest form of vitamin C. It is available as fine crystals, fine powder or in tablet form. One gram equals one fourth of a level teaspoon of the crystals or powder and you can stir it into a glass of juice or into water with honey added. Or you may take it in tablet form, available in 250, 500 or 1,000 mg dosages. It is also available in timed-release capsules which release the vitamin C gradually during an eight-hour period.

Since vitamin C loses strength on prolonged exposure to air or to light, it's important to use only a freshly-opened bottle. Thus it seems best to buy vitamin C in small, opaque jars and to store it in a cool, dark place.

One reason why vitamin C cannot be stored in the body is that plain ascorbic acid is water-soluble. However, a fat-soluble variety, ascorbyl palmitate, is now available. Since body cells have both fat- and water-soluble components, taking a mixture of both fat- and water-soluble ascorbic acid appears to offer some advantages. A recommended mix is one part of ascorbyl palmitate with ten parts of plain ascorbic acid.

Manufactured vitamin C is chemically identical to natural vitamin C. Some plant sources, such as rose hips, have a high concentration of vitamin C but it is chemically identical to the cheapest ascorbic acid.

To minimize irritation, vitamin C is also available in the form of mineral complexes. For instance, people in whom ascorbic acid may cause an excess of stomach acid can take vitamin C buffered with sodium (sodium ascorbate) which neutralizes the acid. For those who must also watch sodium intake, vitamin C is available buffered with calcium (calcium ascorbate).

When mixed with enzymes and stomach acid, ascorbic acid becomes a reactive agent which may not be completely absorbed into the bloodstream. Timed-release capsules overcome this problem. Only twenty per cent or so is dissolved while the capsule is in the stomach. The remainder is timed to be carried into the small intestine where it is absorbed directly into the intestinal wall. Timed-release capsules are available containing either plain ascorbic acid or one of its mineral complexes. Since mineral complexes pass more freely through cell membranes, they are particularly useful to older people whose intestinal cells may have lost some of their ability to absorb nutrients.

Among the various ascorbic acid complexes are calcium ascorbate, manganese ascorbate, zinc ascorbate and magnesium ascorbate. Calcium ascorbate is regarded as highly absorbable and it also aids in relaxing muscles and inducing sleep. The effect of zinc ascorbate on colds appears not to have been tested.

Vitamin C may be neutralized or destroyed in the body by heavy emotional stress, by taking aspirin or the Pill, by smoking or drinking alcohol, by taking procaine or antihistamine, by heavy metal deposits in the body, during recovery from a wound, or during a bacterial invasion. Should one or more of these circumstances coincide with a cold, you might consider moderately increasing your intake of vitamin C.

For example, vitamin C is consumed rapidly while under stress. A study by J. Aleo, D.D.S, Ph.D., and Harish Padh, Ph. D., of Temple University, Philadelphia, has revealed that endotoxin, a natural product of invading bacteria, blocks absorption of vitamin C into the body during a bacterial infection. Under such circumstances, it would appear prudent to increase one's intake of vitamin C moderately, both in the diet and in supplement form.

Conversely, some women have demonstrated the ability to abort a cold if caught within one to two days prior to the beginning of their menstrual period. This ability is believed to be due to a hormone released into the bloodstream. Hence, during the one to two days preceding menstruation, women may require a lower dosage of vitamin C to fight a cold.

However much you may personally decide to increase your vitamin C intake, it's well to resist the temptation to take megadoses. One reason is that when large doses of vitamin C are suddenly stopped, the level of immunocompetence may fall so dramatically that malignant tumors have been observed to grow more rapidly.

Megadoses of vitamin C undoubtedly have some potential for causing discomfort. Diarrhea is the most common complication. It has been suggested that diarrhea can be avoided by changing to a different variety of vitamin C.

Large doses of Vitamin C have also been observed to inhibit the speed and motility of intestinal muscle movement, causing stomach gas. This discomfort can usually be reduced by cutting down on meat, poultry, fried foods and beans. Cutting down on these same foods may also reduce incidence of heartburn associated with vitamin C. Some observers have reported that, in any case, vitamin C-associated heartburn will disappear spontaneously by the third day. It may also be reduced by taking an alkalizer.

According to Linus Pauling, ascorbic acid will not

affect ulcers nor cause kidney stones. If you are prone to kidney stone formation, however, you could reduce the risk by using sodium ascorbate or by taking ascorbic acid with an alkalizer.

The vitamin C doses suggested in this chapter should be restricted to full-grown adults of normal body size. For use in children under 100 pounds body weight, dosages should be reduced in proportion to body weight. However, holistic vitamin C therapy is not recommended for children owing to the difficulty of getting them to take the regular dosages.

A final caveat: if you experience adverse side effects due to taking vitamin C for a cold or flu, we strongly recommend that you cease taking further dosages. However, in the relatively small amounts suggested here, it is extremely unlikely that you will experience any discomfort. We also recommend that if you are taking prescription medication or are undergoing medical treatment or supervision of any type of dysfunction, that you consult your physician before using vitamin therapy of any kind, including vitamin A and zinc gluconate tablets.

Vitamin E

Preliminary studies have suggested that moderate amounts of vitamin E (in the range of 200 IU per day) assist phagocytes in destroying pathogenic invaders. In contrast, a deficiency of vitamin E has been found to diminish antibody production and to inhibit lymphocyte proliferation in response to a non-self antigen.

Vitamin E is an antioxidant, meaning it has a powerful capacity to neutralize free radicals (stray electrons which can reactively damage the genetic nucleus of body cells). Several studies have shown that in enhancing immunocompetence, vitamin E works synergistically with other antioxidants such as vitamin C and the mineral selenium.

It has also been observed that megadoses of vitamin E have had the opposite effect. They have inhibited immunocompetence and in some cases, they have increased blood pressure. For this reason, many nutritionists suggest a daily maintenance dose of 100 IU of vitamin E during the cold season. During a cold, this can be increased to 200 IU, returning to the 100 IU dosage some two weeks later. It has also been suggested that during a cold, older people could take up to 400 IU per day because of poorer absorption potential. This amount should not be maintained for more than 14 days.

It is important to be certain that you are taking vitamin E only in the form of d-alpha or dl-alpha tocopherol. Other varieties such as beta, delta or gamma tocopherol offer fewer benefits. For best absorption, the acetate form of alpha tocopherol is often preferred.

Iron

A deficiency of iron has been observed to cause a wide variety of defects in immune system function. However, too much iron can aid bacterial invaders in multiplying. The suggested daily intake is 25 mg during a cold and 20 mg otherwise.

Magnesium

Magnesium dilates arteries and relaxes muscles throughout the body, thereby inducing a feeling of calm. This serenity, in turn, helps to enhance immunocompetence. All evidence suggests that an adequate magnesium intake is essential for keeping arteries relaxed and for remaining at ease during the stress of a cold or flu infection. The recommended daily intake is 500 mg during a cold and 400 mg otherwise.

Zinc

When a three-year-old child with leukemia was given a zinc gluconate tablet to restore a zinc deficiency, and to stimulate her immune system, she accidentally discovered a rapid way to end the common cold.

Because she had a sore throat, the child sucked on the zinc gluconate tablet instead of swallowing it and she allowed it to dissolve in her mouth. The sore throat was due to an endless series of colds the child had suffered, and the zinc was prescribed because she had just come down with symptoms of yet another cold. Curiously, however, instead of turning into another full-blown cold, within twelve hours her cold symptoms had vanished altogether.

Impressed, the child's father carried out the same therapy on other family members as they caught colds. He also repeated it the next time the leukemic child caught a cold. In nearly every case, cold symptoms disappeared within twelve to twenty-four hours.

Two years later a study was authored by Dr. William Halcomb, an Austin, Texas family practitioner. Reportedly, a total of 146 people, all of whom had had a viral cold for three days or less, took either a 180 mg zinc gluconate lozenge (containing 22 mg of essential zinc) or a placebo.

They began by initially taking two tablets, then every two hours during the waking day, they took another 180 mg zinc gluconate lozenge. Not more than twelve tablets were taken in any one day. Each subject was instructed to hold the lozenge in the mouth for ten minutes until it had completely dissolved *and not to chew or swallow it*. In this way, the zinc saturated the lining of the mouth, tongue and throat. The test subjects kept taking the lozenges at this same rate until all cold symptoms had vanished. But no one was permitted to continue taking these amounts of zinc for more than seven days.

Results were quite dramatic: 11 percent of the zinc-treated group lost all cold symptoms within twelve hours; 22 percent were cold-free in twenty-four hours; 50 percent were cold-free in about four days; and 88 percent were cold-free in seven days. By comparison, all of the placebo group still had cold symptoms after four days; and only 49 percent were cold-free by the seventh day. On balance, the zinc-treated group shortened the duration of cold symptoms by seven days. Results were the same whether a person had a mild or a severe cold.

These conclusions resulted from an analysis of the double blind study by the Clayton Foundation Biochemical Institute at the University of Texas, Austin, Texas. Dr. Donald Davis, Ph. D., of the Clayton Foundation reportedly suggested that zinc ions might inhibit cleavage of viral polypeptides thus preventing replication of viruses inside nasal cells. Study results were published in *Antimicrobial Agents and Chemotherapy Journal*, January 1984.

But some subjects reported that the zinc tablets distorted their taste and caused stomach upset. Others experienced nausea when taking the lozenges on an empty stomach. Should vomiting or other intestinal distress occur, you should immediately cease taking the zinc lozenges. Zinc therapy for children is best undertaken only under a physician's directions.

Although test subjects in the Texas study were reported to have been given 180 mg zinc gluconate tablets, here again the zinc was given alone with no mention of additional supportive nutrition such as vitamins A, C and E. Since 50 mg zinc gluconate lozenges with a natural orange flavor are available in most health food stores, we suggest using the 50 mg lozenge for "holistic zinc therapy," meaning that you take it in conjunction with the full spectrum of other supportive nutrients recommended in this chapter.

Although the 50 mg zinc lozenges contain only seven mgs of essential zinc, in conjunction with all other supportive nutrients this would appear to give you an adequate supply of zinc. By taking one 50 mg zinc gluconate lozenge every two hours while awake, you should not experience any of the discomfort reported in the Texas study.

Although the dosages suggested in that study appear to have been endorsed by physicians, other doctors have cautioned that these amounts are quite high and should certainly not be continued for more than a week. We also strongly urge that treatment with the 50 mg zinc gluconate lozenges should also not be extended beyond seven days. Taking zinc for a longer period may cause toxicity and actually lower immunocompetence. For routine maintenance, 25 mg of zinc gluconate per day (or of zinc in any other form) is considered adequate during the cold season and 15 mg during the remainder of the year.

In recent years, numerous other studies have documented that a zinc deficiency will contribute to immunosuppression, including atrophy of lymphoid tissue and abnormalities in both T and B cells. A significant proportion of elderly Americans is believed to be deficient in zinc. Researchers have shown that when an adequate zinc intake is restored, immune system function swiftly responds by increasing the number of T lymphocytes and increasing sensitivity to antigens.

By way of proof, Patricia Wagner, Ph. D. coauthored a study at the University of Florida, relating zinc levels to overall immune response in 203 subjects aged sixty to ninety-three. Tests showed that forty-five persons had weakened immune systems, and these same people all had the lowest zinc levels. When five of these subjects were given fifty-five mg of zinc daily for four weeks, their immuno-competence was restored.

However, it was concluded that most people need only 15 mg of zinc daily to ensure immunocompetence. Those who eat a variety of vegetables and whole grains may not need supplementation.

In a similar study in Brussels, (reported in the *American Journal of Medicine*, May 1981) Dr. Jean duChateau divided thirty subjects aged seventy and over into two groups. One group took 220 mg of zinc sulphate twice daily for a month and the control group received none. Results showed a significant improvement in a number of immune system components in the zinc-treated group, especially in the number of circulating T cells. This plainly indicates that zinc stimulates the biological activity of white blood cells.

Other studies have confirmed that a zinc deficiency can inhibit the healing of wounds and can reduce activity of the thymus gland, a key factor in T cell production. A deficiency of zinc can also lead to depression, insomnia or anxiety, emotional states which also contribute to immuno-suppression.

Summing Up

The massive build-up of white blood cells and anti-bodies needed to overcome a viral infection can occur only when suficient vitamins A, C and E, the B complex, zinc and other essential nutrients are present. There is consid-erable evidence that megadoses of a single nutrient, such as vitamin C or zinc, achieve no greater result than more moderate amounts. For optimal benefit, most evidence seems to support a more holistic form of nutritional ther-apy based on taking the smaller amounts of essential nutrients recommended in this chapter. Since no study has been made using a holistic nutritional approach, we cannot say with certainty how swiftly your cold is likely to disappear.

But every indication is that cold symptoms should vanish more rapidly than by using a single nutrient such as vitamin C or zinc. The smaller amounts of each nutrient should also eliminate any risk of intestinal or other discomfort. However, if you do experience any adverse effects due to supplementation, you should cease taking the supplements until you can identify the specific nutrient that is responsible.

6 The Herbal Approach

According to the World Health Organization, herbal products still provide primary health care for 80 percent of the world's population. Even in the U.S., some $8 billion is spent every year on plant-derived medications.

Many plants contain chemicals that have been scientifically validated for use in OTC and prescription drugs. Pharmaceutical companies frequently search among herbs for new drug sources.

Herbs, of course, are widely used in homeopathic medicine. Homeopathy is a healing system in which naturally-occurring herbs and other substances are used to stimulate immunocompetence and other body defense systems. A homeopathic physician uses a patient's symptoms to make a "symptom profile." He then matches it with a medicine having a similar profile—implying that the medicine has produced similar symptoms in a large number of patients.

Most cold or flu symptoms are produced by the body's

defensive reaction to the virus rather than by the virus itself. Hence homeopathy treats the host rather than the virus. Specifically, a homeopathic physician will treat the host's underlying basic vulnerabilty, which translates into enhancing the immune system and other body defenses which may have been weakened.

Only a homeopathic physician has the skill to match a cold sufferer's "symptom profile" with a medication having similar properties. However, if you have access to a homeopathic physician and your cold or flu is severe enough to warrant homeopathic intervention, you will find a wide range of natural remedies available.

Although many of them may be prescribed only by a homeopathic doctor, many other common herbal remedies can provide soothing relief from colds, flu and other respiratory disorders. A brief rundown of those most highly favored by herbalists follows.

The favored way to take most herbs is in the form of a tea. Simply make a fairly strong brew, equivalent to suffusing one tea bag of black tea in a cup of boiling water. However, some herbs such as cinnamon, garlic, pepper, mustard and radish may also be taken in food. Under no circumstances try to smoke herbs to clear congestion or to relieve any other respiratory symptoms. Regardless of its source, smoke is a harsh irritant that will inhibit cilia action and inflame the mucous membranes.

General Cold Remedies

Cut up two lemons and steep in a pot of boiling water for twelve to fifteen minutes. Serve with a tablespoon of honey added to each cup. Alternatively, squeeze the juice from a large lemon and mix into a small glass of warm water. Sip slowly. Herbalists claim that as components in the lemon juice oxidize, ozone is released which enhances immunocompetence. Whether or not this is so, the citric acid works beneficially to increase the acid level of mucosa in the throat.

Herbal remedies for preventing colds and flu are available in many health food stores. They are believed to work by enhancing immunocompetence. Herbs commonly used in these formulas include Flos lonicerae, Echinacea, Fructus forsythia, Siberian Ginseng and Radix astragalus.

Lavender (Lavendula) is reputed by many herbalists to raise the white blood cell count and to help prevent complications such as pneumonia.

Although we have no scientific confirmation of Garlic's cold-fighting properties, it was used as a cold remedy in Europe until after World War II. It is probably best taken by eating a clove of raw Garlic every three hours, starting immediately a cold begins. Or you could take a capsule of Garlic oil. Although odor-free varieties are available, most herbalists prefer either a natural clove or plain Garlic oil. The odor disappears after 24 hours or so. Garlic is an effective decongestant and expectorant.

A good general cold and flu remedy is Echinacea extract, a herbal preparation made from prairie cornflower. It is best taken in tablet form. Echinacea tablets, combined with vitamin C, are available in most health food stores. Herbalists also often recommend Echinacea for relief of nasal congestion, muscular aches and pains, runny nose and sore throat.

Antihistamines

Widley used in Hindu Ayurvedic medicine to relieve nasal congestion and post-nasal drip are three herbs which provide a similar effect to antihistamine. They are: Peppermint (Mentha piperita), Anise (Pimpinella anisum) and Ginger (Zingiber officinale).

Bronchodilators

Among efficient natural bronchodilators is black tea (Thea sinensis) which contains theophylline, the favorite medical drug for asthma relief. While black tea contains only a mild amount of theophylline, its caffeine content will also help to open up congested sinuses. Black tea also makes a good expectorant and a fairly strong cup containing a teaspoon of lemon juice will give you a lift that makes cold symptoms feel better under almost any circumstances.

Among other effective natural bronchodilators are Ma Huang (Ephedra sinica). You may take it as a tea or in tablet form, available in most health food stores. It is also a popular hayfever remedy. Because Ma Huang is a stimulant that raises blood pressure and pulse rate, it should not be taken continuously.

Chest Rubs

Natural chest rubs help stimulate circulation in the chest and lung area while their vapors also help relieve nasal congestion. You can make a good chest rub by mixing together equal amounts of thymol, menthol, Eucalyptus oil, myristica oil, turpentine oil and Cedarleaf oil.

Another chest rub formula is to mix two to three drops each of Peppermint and Eucalyptus plus essential oil of either Lavender or Rosemary (or both) into one-fourth cup of olive oil. Rub the mixture well into the chest and cover with a warm cloth. Inhale the vapors.

Cough Suppressants

While no natural cough remedy will entirely suppress the brain's cough center, a variety of herbal remedies will effectively soothe a cough by providing relief for a sore or itchy throat.

A tea made of Comfrey (Symphytum officinale) provides lasting relief for a persistent cough. For a dry, nonproductive cough, try a tea made of Coltsfoot (Tussilago farfara).

However, three herbs are claimed to at least partially suppress the brain's cough center. Anise will diminish the most hacking cough to where it is no longer irritating. Eucalyptus (Eucalyptus globulus) and Peppermint are also effective natural cough suppressants.

Menthol lozenges work locally in the throat area to relieve symptoms of cough and sore throat. Only a single lozenge should be taken each hour.

Licorice (Glycyrrhiza glabra) also provides soothing relief for a sore throat. It is popular with asthma and hayfever sufferers because of its ability to stimulate the adrenal glands in event of adrenal exhaustion. Since licorice may raise blood pressure, it should be used sparingly by those with hypertension.

Slippery Elm lozenges, available in almost all health food stores, bring blessed comfort to those afflicted with a sore throat. Slippery Elm (Ulmus falva) is made by grinding the inner bark of the tree into a fine powder. The herb also has a high nutritional content of iron and calcium.

Decongestants

A weak tea made of Cayenne powder (red pepper) makes an effective nasal decongestant and is a favorite with sinus sufferers. Also available at health food stores in capsules, cayenne will swiftly break up and remove mucus congestion. It is also a splendid cough reliever.

Ma Huang tea, previously mentioned, is also an effective sinus decongestant.

But perhaps the most effective of all natural decongestants is the old fashioned steam inhaler. Make a dish of tea
out of essential oils of Eucalyptus, Rosemary, Juniper,
Pine and Rose Geranium—or out of as many as you can
obtain. Have the dish simmering on the stove. Place the
dish on a plate or in a pan and put on a table. Lean over
the dish, keep the eyes closed, cover the head with a
towel, and inhale the richly-flavored vapor into the nasal
passages, sinuses and lungs. It will swiftly break up any
congestion.

If unable to obtain the other oils, Eucalyptus oil alone
makes an effective steam inhalant. Recent lab studies have
shown that Eucalyptus, black pepper and cinnamon have
an inhibitory effect on influenza viruses A1 and A2. Cinnamon and black pepper may be taken with food.

Expectorants

Since the FDA Advisory Review Panel was unable to
find any effective OTC expectorants, most people are discovering that natural substances are much to be preferred.
Water thins secretions in the throat and lungs so that it
can be coughed up more easily. Water is best taken in the
form of hot soups. Vegetable soups are especially good for
thinning mucus and increasing fluid in the respiratory
tract. Onion soup is considered superior to the much-
vaunted chicken soup. In any case, be sure to keep your
air passages clear by drinking plenty of warm teas and
soups.

Among effective herbal expectorants are Wild Cherry
bark (Prunus serotina) or Gumweed (Grindelia robusta).
Used as a tea, either will relax muscle spasms in the lungs
and reduce coughing. Mullein (Verbascum thapsus) is
another popular expectorant which, herbalists claim, also
soothes swollen throat glands and inflamed tissue.

Freshly-squeezed, undiluted Lemon juice is another powerful expectorant, if taken a teaspoon at a time mixed with a little honey.

Pepper, Mustard, Garlic and Radish are other expectorants. A study made at UCLA found that when enough of these condiments were eaten to cause tingling in the tongue and cheeks, and running of the nose and sneezing, one is taking the optimal amount for expectorant purposes. The best varieties are Black Pepper (Piper nigrum), Horseradish (Armoriacia lapathifolia), Garlic (Allium sativum), Chili Pepper (Capsicum species) and Mustard (Brassica species). They are best taken as small amounts to flavor food.

Licorice is also a good expectorant and is also often used to relieve smoker's cough. A tea of Fenugreek or Mullein works well as an expectorant. Mullein also appears to have painkilling properties while it also serves to calm the nerves.

Most natural expectorants are available as teas, tinctures, tablets or in syrup form. To make a really efficient expectorant tea, mix together equal parts of Mullein, Comfrey leaf, Licorice, Coltsfoot and Elecampane (Inula helenium). This five-combination tea is also an effective decongestant, a bronchodilator and a cough reliever. Several herbalists have recommended taking up to six cups of this tea per day as a general cold remedy. Children may be given proportionately smaller amounts.

The above formula can also be made into a cough syrup. Use three teaspoons of the mixture to brew a strong cup of tea, strain it and mix with a teaspoon of honey. You will then have produced a tasty syrup which can be sipped throughout the day.

Fever Reduction

A popular homeopathic remedy that relieves fever by stimulating sweating is a tea made of Hyssop (Hyssopus officinalis) or Boneset (Eupatorium perfoliatum). A mix of the two will combine the decongestant qualities of Hyssop with the pain-relieving properties of Boneset.

Mucilage

Herbs that coat the air passages and throat with a soothing coat of mucilage are favorites with herbalists. Worthy of mention in this respect are cod liver oil and Garlic oil, either of which coat the mucosa of the throat and bronchial passages and relieve soreness and coughing. Cod liver oil is also an important source of vitamins A and D.

Mullein also works effectively as a mucilage, its pain-killing qualities helping to calm the nerves and to sooth inflamed tissue. Ginger root, used either as a gargle or a tea, is a traditional mucilage that soothes inflamed mucous membranes.

Another popular Ginger recipe is this. Heat a small pan of low-fat milk, being careful not to boil it. Add half a teaspoon of ground ginger or two to three slices of fresh Ginger. Served with honey, this makes a soothing mucilage that will coat and protect the throat and larynx.

Comfrey leaves and roots are another popular source of mucilage for upper respiratory tract ailments. Herbalists often recommend Comfrey to asthma sufferers.

Another splendid mucilage can be made from Slippery Elm. Place a heaping teaspoon of powdered Slippery Elm bark in a bowl and mix into a paste with cold water. Next, keep stirring as you slowly add a cup of boiling water. Smooth out any lumps with an egg beater. To take this mucilage, mix it with cow's milk or soy milk, and sip.

Sedatives

Natural sedatives can help calm both body and mind, thereby stimulating the biological activity of the immune system. Natural sedatives most often recommended by herbalists include Catnip (Nepeta cataria) which is particularly helpful for relaxing nerves in the chest and lung area. Others include Skullcap (Scutellaria lateriflora), Hops (Humulus lupulus) and Valerian (Valeriana officinalis). All should be taken in very moderate amounts. Chamomile tea is another efficient relaxant which can be drunk without restriction.

Herbal pocket inhalers are available in many health food stores. Alternatively, you may place one or more essential oils in a humidifier or vaporizer. The vapors will soon permeate your home and will work constantly to soothe cold symptoms.

Almost all of the herbs and herbal remedies mentioned in this chapter can be found in the herb departments of larger health food stores. The majority are also carried by almost all medium-sized health food stores. It is important to realize that although available without prescription, some of these herbs are quite powerful and they should be used sparingly. Discontinue immediately the use of any which appear to cause adverse effects.

7 The Physical Approach

Probably the most useful of all physical techniques is the ability to recognize the early warning signs of an impending cold.

These signs frequently precede onset of a cold by up to twelve hours. They are: the nose and throat feel dry and tight; and mild, tickling sensation exists in the throat; you feel less hungry than normal; and you may also have a mild feeling of being slightly below par.

As soon as these signs become clearly discernible, begin doing everything possible to retard progress of the cold and to build up immunocompetence.

Stop smoking and drinking alcohol. Begin drinking extra fluids such as water, juices, soups and teas. Minimize your upcoming schedule and work load. Stay calm and relaxed and avoid stress. Take a brisk walk, if you can, to stimulate the immune system. But after that, stay rested and conserve energy. Go to bed early, remain warm and comfortable, and study Chapters 8 and 9. If you don't have to go to work, rest and recuperate at home.

Here, one by one, is a review of other physical steps we can take to relieve cold symptoms, to make ourselves feel better and more comfortable, and to shorten the duration of the infection.

Stop Sunbathing

New research on photo-immunology has revealed that exposing the body to intense sunlight for an hour or more at a time—as while sunbathing—can suppress the immune system for as long as fifteen days.

Immuno-suppression occurs because 15 percent of the blood is constantly in the capillaries of the skin where solar radiation may easily damage lymphocytes. This phenomenon is easily proved by the fact that many people who sunbathe in strong sunlight for periods of an hour or more frequently experience fever blisters on the mouth shortly afterwards. These blisters are caused by Herpes Simplex Virus #1 which can emerge only when the immune system is suppressed.

For the same reason, people often come down with a cold or flu after sunbathing. So if you're planning a mid-winter beach vacation in the Caribbean or Mexico, be sure to take along plenty of sunscreen block.

Stop Smoking

Smoking not only increases your risk of catching a viral infection but it also intensifies the symptoms and prolongs the duration. Worse still, it triples the risk of a complication.

To begin with, irritants in tobacco smoke paralyze the cilia, the hair-like cells that sweep invading viruses out of the nasal passages. As a result, a smoker runs twice the risk of catching a cold as does a nonsmoker.

Smoking also seriously impairs immunocompetence. Among many studies confirming this fact was a recent Australian investigation which found that smokers had below-normal levels of killer T cells. However, six weeks after some of the subjects in the study decided to quit smoking, their levels of killer T cells began to increase. In a few months, normal levels were restored.

Other studies have shown that smoking reduces the beneficial effects of vitamin C and other essential nutrients by at least forty per cent.

Hence you should stop smoking completely at the first sign of a cold. If you can refrain from smoking for the duration of a cold or flu attack, you may decide to quit altogether.

Exercise Briskly Every Day

Ever since oncologist O. Carl Simonton, M.D. noted that cancer patients who exercised had a significantly higher recovery rate than those who did not, new evidence has been emerging to prove that exercise enhances immuno-competence.

For example, researchers in athletic medicine have noted a clear relationship between regular physical exercise and a decreased risk of infection. Incidence of cancer in active people is significantly lower than in sedentary people.

In another study, researchers at both Purdue University and the University of Arizona, in studying the combined effects of vitamins C and E plus exercise, found that vigor-ous exercise enhanced the vitamins' immunity-building properties. They also discovered that people who exercised and did *not* take supplements still had appreciably higher levels of T lymphocytes.

Indications are also emerging to show that exercise stimulates activity of macrophages and lymphocytes. Regular daily physical exercise has also been observed to increase levels of lymphokine 1 and interferon, both of which strengthen immunocompetence.

Some researchers believe this is because soon after exercise is begun, the adrenals secrete epinephrine and norepinephrine, neurotransmitters which increase the body's metabolic rate by as much as 100 percent. Part of this overall stimulation is to increase immune system activity. Epinephrine also constricts nasal blood vessels, causing nasal membranes to shrink and air passages to open up. Thus exercise makes breathing much easier during a cold.

Exercise has also been observed to stimulate the brain to produce painkilling endorphins and enkephalins. Together with epinephrine and norepinephrine, they raise the pain threshold, thereby easing the discomfort of cold symptoms. They also reduce anxiety and create a powerful feeling of wellbeing.

Additionally, exercise has been demonstrated to stimulate release of pyrogen by the immune system. This chemical messenger raises the body's core temperature slightly above normal for several hours. In the process, the nose temperature is also increased to above its normal high of 95°F. Since cold viruses have difficulty in maintaining biological activity at temperatures above 95°, millions of viral invaders tend to shrivel up and become inactive. Exercise also helps a person relax and sleep during an infection.

While you should certainly not exercise with a fever, nor at any time you do not feel like it, nonetheless the benefits of a brisk walk are plainly obvious. A brisk three to five mile daily walk during a cold should not only shorten the duration but also help keep nasal passages clear, and reduce the severity of other symptoms.

Regular daily exercise throughout the year should produce even greater benefits. Any kind of continuous, rhythmic exercise such as brisk walking, race walking, jogging, brisk bicycling, swimming, aerobic dancing or calisthenics should enhance immunocompetence on a permanent basis. When and if a cold is caught, the immune system is much better prepared to launch a counterattack.

By exercising regularly throughout the year, you can maintain a level of fitness that will enable you to continue exercising during a cold. Any recommendation to exercise naturally assumes that you are sufficiently fit to undertake the exercise without fatigue or any other risk to your health. If you are not accustomed to regular daily exercise, you should not suddenly begin to exercise vigorously when you have caught a cold. Older persons, smokers, those who are overweight, or anyone with a chronic disease or dysfunction, or who is under medical treatment, should consult a physician before beginning to exercise.

However, if you are in normally sound health, you should be able to take a brisk daily walk without risk to your health.

Keep the Mucous Membranes Moist

When the mucous lining of the membranes in the nose and throat dry out, they fail to trap invading viruses. Dry air also immobilizes the cilia which sweep trapped viruses into the stomach for destruction. Especially if your vocal cords are affected, or if you have laryngitis or a sore throat, you should try to avoid breathing very dry air.

During winter, many homes in the north are heated to high tempratures which cause the humidity to reach extremely low levels. This condition encourages viral infections.

The simplest way to raise the humidity indoors is to lower the temperature a few degrees. However, a humidifier or vaporizer provides an effective way to prevent the mucous membranes from drying out. Failing this, humidity can be restored by keeping a kettle of water simmering on a low burner. By placing a few drops of eucalyptus oil, or other essential oil, in a humidifier or vaporizer, you can create a pleasing vapor that will help soothe cold symptoms.

How to Blow Your Nose Correctly

Never blow the nose vigorously and try to avoid closing one nostril while blowing. That can create extra pressure in the other nostril, forcing mucus into the Eustachian tube and possibly causing a middle ear infection.

Instead, the nose should be blown gently, softly and repeatedly with both nostrils left free and unprotected. Avoid sniffling because of the ease with which viruses can be sniffed into the sinuses.

Try to keep the jaw relaxed while blowing your nose.

How to Stop Nosebleed

In dry winter air, nasal membranes tend to dry out and crack. Thus blood vessels may bleed during vigorous nose blowing.

To stop a nosebleed, pinch the nostrils tightly for ten minutes or until a blood clot has formed. If you know in which nostril the bleeding is occurring, you need only close that side.

Alternatively, you can roll up a small wad of cotton wrapped in gauze, or you can use ordinary paper tissue, and use this to loosely plug the nostril. Remove it after ten minutes. Care must then be taken not to blow your nose again for at least twelve hours.

How to Clear a Blocked Nose

If one nostril seems completely blocked, dissolve half a teaspoon of salt in a glass of warm (but not hot) water. Insert the nose into the glass and suck up water through the unblocked nostril. Keep sucking up water until you feel it run down the back of your throat. Then remove the glass and allow the water to drain out of the nose. Blow the nose gently and steadily into a tissue. Repeat several times, if necessary, to unblock the nasal passage. The water will flush out excess mucus without irritating mucous membranes. You can repeat this natural decongestant four or five times a day.

Relieving Sinus or Ear Pain

A sharp pain in the ear during a cold may indicate an ear infection. Try to stop sniffling and blow your nose very gently. The pain can usually be relieved by applying a heating pad to the ear. However, if pain persists, see a physician without delay.

Sinus discomfort may also often be relieved by applying a heating pad to the painful area. If persistent pain occurs on the surface or forehead, see a physician.

How to Feel Comfortable Quickly

Assuming you do not have a fever, take a long relaxing soak in a hot tub bath. If only a shower is available, run the water as hot as possible over each part of your body but especially the back and shoulders and the back of the neck. Pour a teaspoon of lemon juice into a cup of black tea or, if you prefer, a herb tea such as chamomile or peppermint. Then rest in a warm bed, sip the tea and read a good book. Or read Chapter 9 of this book. Continue to drink plenty of fluids.

If your infection turns out to be flu (see symptoms in Chapter 3 under heading "How to tell whether you have a cold or influenza") you should remain in bed for as long as your temperature stays above normal. Resting in bed allows the body to focus its energy on the healing process while getting up might lead to a complication. You can safely take a sponge bath while in bed. But don't get up to bathe or shower. After your temperature returns to normal, you should remain at home for an extra day and resume normal activities gradually.

If you feel the need to reduce fever, you can do so by taking an alcohol bath. However, fever is usually part of the healing process.

Inhaling Steam

Already mentioned under the heading "Decongestants" in Chapter 6, steam combined with herbal vapors makes a very effective decongestant. But steam does more than merely free blocked nasal air passages. It heats up the nose, making it too hot for viruses to thrive.

Both flu and cold viruses flourish in a temperature of 86° to 96°F. Since the body's core temperature is 98.6°, the body itself is too hot for these viruses to inhabit. But the temperature of nasal air passages is closer to the virus's comfort range. During a severe viral infection, the immune system secretes pyrogen, a chemical messenger which triggers the brain's temperature control to raise body temperature to about 102°. As the overall temperature increase spreads to the nose, the nasal membranes become uncomfortably hot and millions of viruses become biologically inactive. This is one way in which fever aids the healing process.

Another way to make the nose untenably hot for viruses is by inhaling steam. Simply heat a dish of water until it is steaming, and then place it on a table. Sit down and lean over the dish, close the eyes, drape a towel over the head, and inhale the steam into the nose, sinuses and lungs.

The steam will soon relieve any congestion. But continue to inhale steam into the nasal passages for as long as you can without discomfort.

Inhaling steam is even more effective and pleasant if you add a few drops of essential oils of Eucalyptus, Rosemary, Juniper, Pine and Rose Geranium. A single one will do but all five are better.

Half an hour is probably the maximum for which anyone would elect to inhale steam. Inhaling steam for ten to fifteen minutes or so each morning and evening can provide wonderful relief for a head cold.

Gargling to Soothe a Raw, Scratchy Throat

Gargling with salt water will provide temporary relief for a raw, scratchy throat. Dissolve half a teaspoon of salt in an eight-ounce glass of warm-to-mildly hot water. Throw the head well back as you gargle, being careful not to swallow.

Another gargle formula is to mix together equal parts of honey and apple cider vinegar in a cup of mildly hot water. This is a traditional folk remedy for relieving congestion.

Commercial gargles containing phenol or benzocaine may temporarily relieve a sore throat.

Relieving Cold Symptoms with Acupressure

To practice this ancient Japanese healing therapy, place both thumbs, nails up, parallel on the table. Now press gently but firmly while making a rotating motion with the thumbs. Hold the pressure for eight seconds, then release. When you apply this to any part of the body, you are practicing acupressure.

To relieve cold symptoms, begin by applying pressure to the center of your forehead directly above the nose. Then, separating the thumbs, begin to press with a single thumb on each side of the bridge of the nose opposite the corner of each eye. Continue working on down the face, next to the nose, at half-inch intervals. You should be massaging with one thumb on each side of the nose, applying pressure for eight seconds in one spot before moving on to the next.

If you find it easier, you may use a fingertip in place of a thumb. Under no circumstances use pressure on the eyes themselves.

Now, using the tips of the third and fourth fingers instead of the thumbs, use the same pressure and motion to massage the top of the head. Then massage the center of the crown and work on down to the back of the neck.

Massaging these key pressure points will invariably bring soothing relief from sinus pain, congestion and headache for periods of thirty to forty-five minutes or more.

8 The Dietary Approach

Can what we eat really help prevent colds and flu and speed recovery? A growing number of studies seem to indicate that the answer is YES.

For example, a report in the *British Medical Journal* (September 1985) describes how researchers in Canada gave flu vaccine to thirty poorly nourished older people, then split them into two groups. The first group was shown how to upgrade their diet with better nutrition and they also received supplements. The second group received nothing. A month later, the nutritionally-improved group showed a significant increase in flu antibodies compared to the control group. The authors felt that better nutrition improved immune response in the fifteen elderly people and gave them stronger protective immunity.

What Is a Good Anti-Cold Diet?

Let's begin with foods to avoid. Topping the list are alcohol and caffeine. Both reduce the benefits of vitamin

C and other essential nutrients by approximately forty per cent while caffeine also causes a zinc deficiency. Beverages containing caffeine include coffee, black and green tea, hot chocolate, cocoa and most cola drinks. The Pill, diuretics, anti-hypertension medication, prescription and "recreational" drugs and medications may also interfere with absorption of nutrients essential to the body's cold-fighting process.

Also ranking high among foods to avoid are fats of all types. A high dietary intake of fat, especially polyunsaturated fatty acids (pressed vegetable oils) and hydrogenated vegetable oils, has been shown to result in lymphoid atrophy and suppressed antibody response to antigens in lab animals. All indications are that fatty acids enhance synthesis of prostaglandins, a surfeit of which are believed to directly suppress the immune system.

However, there are several different types of prostaglandins and certain prostaglandins are utilized by the immune system itself to create inflammation. Prostaglandins are manufactured from linoleic acid, a fatty acid which is transformed into arachidonic acid in the body and is stored in the body's fat cells.

Linoleic acid is supplied by legumes and whole grains such as oatmeal. If, however, you do not eat a sufficiency of these two foods, you can obtain sufficient linoleic acid by adding one teaspoon of cold-pressed sunflower or safflower seed oils to your diet each day. These oils can be used as a dressing on salads or can be used in cooking or in baked goods. (Olive oil or peanut butter are not considered good sources of linoleic acid.) Nonetheless, a single bowl of oatmeal will usually supply our entire linoleic acid needs for the day.

A high-fat diet also inhibits production of "Intrinsic Factor" in the gastric juices which is needed for the absorption of vitamin B12. This nutrient, as you may recall from Chapter 5 is one of a variety of B-complex vitamins which aids the immune system in battling colds and flu. Others include vitamins A, C, E, the entire B-complex and the mineral zinc.

It is foods of animal origin, particularly meat, whole milk dairy products and eggs that are high in fat and low in many vitamins essential to immunocompetence. Refined carbohydrates, such as white flour, sugar and sweeteners of all kinds, are also almost valueless in providing nutritional support. All traces of zinc and other nutrients have been refined out of them. Another problem is that these are all acid-forming foods which interfere with absorption of zinc, and they restrict availability of zinc to the body.

The best nutritional support is provided by eating the 80–10–10 way, meaning that 80 percent of our calories should come from complex carbohydrates (fresh, unprocessed vegetables, fruits, whole grains, nuts, seeds and legumes); not more than ten percent should be derived from fats (preferably from unprocessed fats contained in whole grains, avocados, nuts and seeds); and ten percent should come from protein, preferably from legumes, nuts, seeds, whole grains, white or oily fish, egg whites or very low fat dairy foods such as plain yogurt and cottage cheese.

Eating the 80–10–10 way provides a diet high in vitamins A, C, E and the B-complex and in zinc and most other essential minerals. It also provides sufficient protein for antibody production.

However, it's important that your diet contain an abundance of deep green and yellow vegetables plus green leafy vegetables and both fruits and vegetables which are yellow-to-red or bright orange in color. These foods are all high in beta-carotene, a precursor of vitamin A which is essential to the integrity of mucous membranes lining the nasal air passages.

Disease-Resistant Foods

Among the very best foods you can eat are apricots, cantaloupe, citrus (including lemons and limes), cranberries, mangoes, papaya, peaches, pineapple and strawberries—all good sources of vitamins A and/or C. The best vegetables include asparagus, broccoli, brussels sprouts, carrots, collards, kale, lettuce (excepting iceberg), mustard, pumpkins, sweet pepper, sweet potatoes, winter squash, spinach, turnip greens and most varieties of sprouted seeds and grains—most are also high in vitamins A and C.

Good sources of zinc include plain unbuttered popcorn, sweet potatoes; most nuts, seeds and peanuts; green beans, lentils, wheat germ, wheat bran and brewers or nutritional yeast, which can be sprinkled on cereal. Cod liver oil is also an excellent source of vitamins A and D while most legumes and whole grains supply the B-complex vitamins and vitamin E.

The late Professor Albert Szent-Györgyi, an eminent scientist and Nobel prizewinner, who died recently at the age of 93, reported that since he began eating one-fourth of a cup of wheat germ each day at breakfast several years ago, he did not experience a single cold. Wheat germ is a rich source of zinc as well as vitamin E and manganese.

Because cooking can destroy vitamin C and other vitamins in food, we should eat as many foods as possible fresh and uncooked. For similar reasons, we should avoid all foods that are canned, processed, manufactured, prepared or dehydrated. And when we do cook, we should steam, broil, bake or stew instead of fry.

An important note: dried beans contain zinc but their phytate makes some of that zinc unusable. So be sure to soak the beans overnight before cooking to remove the phytate.

Don't forget, either, that the vitamin C in orange juice, and in other juices, is easily destroyed by freezing, dehydrating or canning. As a result, the actual vitamin C content of most canned or frozen orange and grapefruit juice is often disappointingly low. Whenever possible, either squeeze your own juices from fresh fruits and vegetables; or else eat the fruits and vegetables themselves. Since fruit juices are also high in fruit sugar, which is rapidly absorbed into the bloodstream where it creates a high blood sugar level, fruit juices should be sipped slowly rather than gulped down.

Sparse Eating Helps Colds

Take care not to overeat during a respiratory infection. Overeating causes atrophy of the thymus gland, leading to premature weakening of the immune system.

All T cells are manufactured in the thymus gland which also secretes thymosin, a hormone which orchestrates the growth of the immune system in childhood. During early childhood, the human organism is exposed to a large number of unfamiliar diseases for which antibodies must be formed without delay. But as the teen years approach, antibodies have already been formed for most of the common diseases. Need for thymosin begins to decline and the thymus begins to gradually atrophy. By age sixty, it has declined to approximately one-tenth the size it was in youth. Yet it still plays a vital role in maintaining immunocompetence. All indications thus far are that a frugal diet helps to preserve the size and activity of the thymus gland.

Studies using lab animals at Memorial Sloan-Kettering Cancer Center and at Chase Institute for Cancer Research have all confirmed that frugal eating boosts immunocompetence and reduces incidence of all types of disease and infections. For example, by eating lightly, we can keep the lungs clear and healthy until well into our eight-ies and nineties. The lungs of heavy eaters, by contrast, gradually become filled with cysts and hemorrhaged areas that increase risk of a complication following a cold or flu.

The most recent and important discoveries in this field emanate from the work of Roy C. Walford, Ph.D., an immunologist at UCLA Medical School. Walford has discovered that when calorie intake is gradually reduced by one third while intake of all thirty-two essential vitamins and minerals is maintained, atrophy of the thymus gland is retarded, causing the immune system to remain younger and more active. Put another way, by eating lightly at all times we can, at say age sixty, have an immune system comparable to that of the average person of forty-five.

Thus sparse eating reduces risk of every type of disease including cancer and all respiratory tract infections. We can easily cut calories by reducing such undesirable foods as fats and oils, refined carbohydrates and excessive amounts of animal protein such as meat, whole milk dairy products, and cheeses, ice cream, pizza and eggs. We should also pass up all convenience and fried or fast foods; and all commercial sauces, mayonnaise, dressings and condiments containing fats, oils or sugar. In their place, we can use herbs, lemon juice or garlic to flavor foods.

Eating the 80–10–10 way literally forces us to reduce calorie intake while the fibrous bulk of these complex carbohydrate foods satisfies hunger mechanisms and keeps us feeling full. For instance, fat has 9 calories per gram while protein and refined carbohydrates each have 4. But most complex carbohydrates have only 2.75 calories per gram, less than one-third that of fats. When you consider that 40 percent of the Standard American Diet consists of fat, the high incidence of upper respiratory tract infections is hardly surprising.

Thus the 80–10–10 way of eating not only provides a disease-resistant diet but it will also restore weight to normal.

Diet For Life

Every single study to emerge from modern nutritional science has strongly indicated that our bodies rebel when we eat a diet high in fats, refined carbohydrates and animal protein. Our immune systems, and all other body systems and organs, fare best when we eat a vegetarian diet of complex carbohydrates augmented, if desired, by small amounts of fish, chicken or turkey without the skin, or by low-fat, unflavored yogurt or cottage cheese.

We should also aim to eat as many foods as possible in their primary state, meaning exactly as they exist in nature. Although grains, legumes and tubers may require light cooking, the closer they are to their original natural state, the more they contribute to our being disease-free.

While it helps to eat the 80–10–10 way during an infection, for maximum benefit we should try to follow this way of eating all of the time. Although no controlled study has been made to show that vegetarians have fewer colds, a number of carefully planned studies—including the Framingham study—have clearly demonstrated that vegetarians have a much lower incidence of heart disease, stroke, cancer, hypertension, diabetes, kidney disease, osteoporosis, gallstones and kidney stones, and infectious diseases than do men and women who eat refined carbohydrates and foods of animal origin. It would seem safe, therefore, to extend this list to include the common cold and influenza.

Grandma's Remedies

Recent research suggests that such time-honored remedies as a cup of lemon tea or a bowl of chicken or onion soup may be safer and more effective than many of today's OTC cold medications. These hot beverages, it has been discovered, raise the throat temperature thereby inhibiting viral replication. Furthermore, acid drinks, such as lemon tea or tomato juice, create an acid environment in which the virus cannot exist.

Anyone with a cold or flu should try to drink eight to ten glasses of non-alcoholic liquid during the course of each day. Fluid replacement is especially important during fever when significant loss of body fluids can occur. Among the best drinks are warm, bland soups including onion soup and miso broth, both fruit and vegetable juices—including unsweetened orange, grapefruit, apple or grape juice and also carrot and tomato juice—and carob drinks and teas. Although they contain caffeine, an occasional cup of black or green tea can contribute to the patient's feeling of wellbeing. Try to drink at least half a glass of water or other liquid every half hour.

Foods That Heal

Hot soups act as expectorants by helping loosen secretions from the chest. In our opinion, the very best natural expectorant is a soup made with plenty of onions and garlic simmered in a pot of water with cayenne added.

Tangerines have been found to be effective natural decongestants. In 1960, the Florida Agricultural Experiment Station reported that tangerines contain synephrine, a powerful decongestant. Many people have since reported that a tangerine is more effective than nose drops.

Investigations by Eric Block of the State University of New York at Albany, uncovered the fact that garlic possesses antifungal and antibiotic properties. It was found that garlic contains the chemical allicin which wards off fungi, bacteria and yeast. (Later, allicin turns into ajoene, a substance which inhibits blood clotting and may help prevent a stroke.)

While nothing was found to link garlic with fighting

cold or flu viruses, nonetheless eating garlic raw has long been a traditional folk remedy for colds. Garlic is best taken with foods. Or you can squeeze the oil out of a clove and use it to flavor foods. Alternatively, you can take garlic oil in capsule form. Or you could cut open the capsules and squeeze the oil onto food. Garlic's principal drawback is its unsavory smell.

Plain low-fat yogurt makes a good source of protein and calcium while suffering from an infection. Calcium is essential for metabolism of vitamin C. Yogurt containing *Lactobacillus acidophilus* appears to possess the added property of being able to help heal cold sores and cankers due to herpes simplex virus which may appear on the lips during or after a cold. Acidophilus yogurt is available in most health food stores.

When antibiotics are given to annihilate bacteria during a complication, the antibiotic frequently destroys all or most of the bacterial flora in the digestive tract. Acidophilus yogurt aids in restoring this digestive bacterial flora back to normal.

During the first two days of influenza, adults and children are often unable to eat solid foods. When appetite returns on the third day, it's best to start with a bland diet consisting of soups, steamed vegetables, baked beans and broiled chicken or baked fish.

Finally, any new mother who is wondering whether it's OK to continue to nurse a baby when the mother has a cold, can relax. Most pediatricians concur that a mother can safely continue to nurse an infant. They also advise eating plenty of fruits and not skipping any meals.

9 The Positive Approach

A rapidly expanding reservoir of facts emerging from the leading edge of scientific research is offering intriguing evidence of the mind's healing power.

We now know that the effect of our beliefs, thoughts, emotions and attitudes—including spiritual beliefs—is the largest single influence on the body's health and well-being. Evidence is rapidly accumulating that by letting go of fear, depression and helplessness, and by replacing them with love, hope and other positive emotions, we can bolster immunocompetence and significantly shorten the duration and lessen the impact of a viral infection.

Most of this information has resulted from studies on the link between the immune system and cancer. This is because both cold and flu viruses, and cancer, invoke an almost identical immune response. The same techniques that help the immune system overcome cancer help it to destroy viral infections. And researchers are discovering that psycho-techniques exist through which people are able to overcome terminal cancer.

Back in 1983, for instance, Bill Robertson and Cathie McLeod, both in their fifties, were reportedly undergoing chemotherapy at Scotland's Edinburgh Western General Hospital. Both had been diagnosed as having terminal leukemia and each had been given only a few weeks or months to live.

But while in hospital they met and fell in love. Each immediately began to feel that life was worth living again. Cathie recalls telling herself, "You're going to stay alive," and Bill recalled how he felt new hope surging through his body. Almost immediately, he found himself believing he would beat cancer.

Powered by their new love and hope for the future, both determined to get well. Each made such rapid progress that their leukemias were soon in remission. They got married and, recently, both were still fully recovered and entirely free of cancer.

As a result of this, and hundreds of other documented cases in which terminal cancer patients have completely recovered, the mind-body link is now being seriously explored. Large institutions such as the National Institutes of Health and the Office of Naval Research are funding studies to rigorously test the ways by which our beliefs and thoughts can strengthen or weaken the immune system.

Young Frontier of Immunology

To explore the interface between body, mind and immune system, the new study of psychoneuroimmunology was born. Already, studies in this young discipline have revealed a wealth of exciting information. The existence of an emotional component in cold and flu infections has been identified and researchers have discovered that thinking certain thoughts can bolster our immunocompetence in as short a time as an hour or two. Thus our beliefs and thoughts can influence the duration and severity of a cold or flu, even though we may already be suffering from an infection. In fact, there is increasing evidence to show that our feelings and attitude can do more to speed antibody production than any other single factor.

Numerous studies have already shown that stress, depression, and feeling lonely or helpless suppress the immune system. One recent study found that moderately-stressed or depressed women have 40 percent fewer killer T cells and 20 percent fewer helper T cells than normal.

A similar study of forty-nine medical students made at Ohio State University revealed that their resistance to viral infection was highest after they had spent a vacation relaxing and lowest during the stress of studying for exams. The same study also showed that the loneliest students had less resistance to virus than those who were more gregarious.

Loneliness Lowers Immunocompetence

The role of loneliness in reducing resistance to the common cold was recently demonstrated in England. Researchers recruited fifty-two men and women and classified each as an introvert or an extrovert. All were then inoculated with cold viruses and kept in hospital for ten days of observation. Tests showed that those with extrovert, outgoing personalities had milder cough symptoms while the withdrawn introverts had worse colds. However, the worst colds of all occurred in those who had recently experienced a cluster of stressful life events.

Several other studies, including one recently made at the University of Denver, have also demonstrated that monkeys deprived of contact with their parents or peers, and forced into loneliness, showed significantly decreased levels of T and B cell activity.

It has also been observed that colds and flu—and

particularly pneumonia—commonly occur after one or more stressful life events that cause significant change requiring adaptation. Examples are: divorce, separation, retirement, being fired, and losing a loved one, money or possessions. Anxiety, non-forgiveness, resentment, fear and disappointment, and other negative feelings, are often followed almost immediately by a viral infection. If these negative feelings are prolonged, they may eventually be transformed into cancer.

Feeling helpless has been found to be another powerful immuno-suppressant. Millions of people believe they have no control over their health. They believe that colds and flu strike at random and that nothing can be done to prevent them nor to shorten the duration or lessen the severity of symptoms. Such helplessness has frequently been identified with cancer.

Researchers have discovered that the condition of our immune system exactly mirrors our beliefs, thoughts, feelings and moods and the attitudes we hold about ourselves and others. Whatever we focus our minds on is what we get. The way in which we perceive our strengths, self-worth and competence is translated into our immunocompetence.

Literally dozens of separate studies are strongly confirming that negative beliefs, thoughts, feelings and attitudes suppress immunocompetence while positive beliefs, thoughts, emotions and attitudes enhance immunocompetence.

Role of Emotions in Physical Illness

Researchers have already discovered that we can bolster our immunocompetence by using only positive beliefs and thoughts and by eliminating negative ones. That we can control our immunocompetence through a psycho-technique such as this should come as no surprise. For over twenty years, we have been able to control our arteries and lower blood pressure through a psycho-technique called biofeedback.

Positivism describes the psycho-technique now being used to bolster immunocompetence. It was largely developed out of the pioneering work of medical doctors such as oncologist Bernie Siegel, Herbert Benson and Dean Ornish, all of Harvard Medical School; oncologist O. Carl Simonton M.D.; David T. Burns, M.D., of the University of Pennsylvania; psychiatrist Gerald Jampolsky, M.D., originator of attitudinal healing, and many more.

The sum total of their discoveries is that when we continue to carry fear, guilt, non-forgiveness, resentment, envy, hostility and worry—and when we continue to judge and condemn others—these negative emotions are transformed into pathological changes such as cancer, ulcers, heart disease or infections.

At this stage, we should mention that psychology has long known that every feeling must first be triggered by a thought. A thought, incidentally, is the same thing as creating a mental image or making a mental picture in your mind's eye. Think a thought, or make a mental picture, of a friend or neighbor who has a more exciting spouse, a better job, a bigger house and a more luxurious car than you do, and you've set yourself up for a strong feeling of envy with possible overtones of resentment. Within a minute or two, these negative emotions will start low-grade stress mechanisms simmering and you will begin to feel tense, uncomfortable and upset.

It's not easy to change a negative emotion such as this once it's begun. But it would have been extremely easy to have slid that first thought off your mind when you started comparing yourself with someone else.

If negative thoughts can produce negative emotions

which can be transformed into physiological diseases such as cancer, hypertension and viral infections, then it follows that if we think positive thoughts, we can turn on positive emotions that will bolster our immunocompetence to the point where it can overcome tumors and swiftly produce armies of antibodies to annihilate a viral infection.

We Can Control Our Feelings by Controlling Our Thoughts

Psychologists have discovered that we can feel any way we want to feel at any time by simply thinking an appropriate thought. Should a negative thought intrude on our inner movie screen, we can easily slide it off and replace it with a positive image, such as a beautiful beach or garden scene, before the negative thought can trigger a health-wrecking emotion.

Learning to control our thoughts isn't nearly as difficult as most of us believe. Researchers at the University of Pennsylvania and other university medical schools have completely reversed tens of thousands of cases of severe depression by teaching patients to think positively. Called Cognitive Therapy, it is based on the discovery that most cases of depression are caused not by some complex biological process deep within the body or subconscious mind, but by ten easily recognizable ways in which we distort our thinking by using a negative approach.

It has also been learned that the type of thoughts we get are determined by our beliefs. When we view the world through a filter of negative beliefs we get negative thoughts and feelings. And vice versa. By restructuring our belief system and replacing negative beliefs based on the conditioned past with new, positive beliefs that are more appropriate to the present, we can guarantee ourselves only positive thoughts and feelings.

Positivism simplifies the process of controlling our thoughts by recognizing that all benefits, thoughts and emotions are either Fear-Based or Love-Based.

Fear Destroys the Body's Defenses

When we place our awareness on Fear-Based beliefs and thoughts, our awareness is in the lower or ego-mind level. We are concerned only with *getting* our own self-interests satisfied. This means *getting* security; *getting* enough sex, food and stimulation; and *getting* power through being right, manipulating people, claiming territory or *getting* more possessions, prestige, fame, recognition or achievement. On this low level of consciousness—which is where most people in the world spend most of their time—we are primarily concerned with *getting* rather than giving. All of these positions are based on fear, the fear that there won't be enough to go around, that we won't get our fair share, that our rights may be violated, or that we won't be accorded recognition or prestige. While beliefs and thoughts on this lower level of consciousness may appear to bring temporary pleasure, they almost never produce lasting happiness or satisfaction.

Keeping our awareness on fear-based beliefs and thoughts leads us to think about past memories which trigger either guilt or resentment. Alternatively, we may entertain concern or worries regarding problems that we imagine may confront us in future. We feel constantly threatened and fearful and we make plans to defend ourselves against every contingency that may arise from the hostile, threatening world we perceive around us. We tend to view other people as rivals and our minds are filled with constant chatter as we judge and condemn others.

Amid such chaos, inner peace is impossible. By perceiving everything in our lives through a filter of fear-based beliefs, we see everyone and everything as a threat to our comfort, security and possessions. We feel separated and alone from other people and we are at the mercy of the entire gamut of negative emotions.

These destructive feelings keep our fight or flight response constantly simmering. Our bodies exist in a state of tension and emergency with all systems GO. Glucocorticoid secreted by the adrenal glands shuts down part of the immune system. Blood is also drawn away from the skin and mucosal areas in the nose and throat and directed to the large body muscles instead. When we feel negative, the mouth becomes dry and and the acidity of the nasal mucosa is reduced, lowering our resisting to invading viruses.

How Positivism Heals

Positivism has the opposite effect. When we consciously place our awareness on love-based beliefs and thoughts, we begin to see the world as a loving, friendly, non-threatening place. Our focus is on the immediate here and now. By zeroing in on the present moment, we are able to let go of the past and all its guilts and resentments, and we realize that whatever the future may bring, we are perfectly capable and confident of being able to handle it.

We also discover that we already have everything we need to enjoy the present moment. Hence, right now, at this moment there is nothing we need or want. As a result, we feel content and we begin to experience inner peace. In the process, we suddenly realize we are no longer judging or condemning others. This, in turn, leads us to forgive everyone whom we once believed had harmed us in some way.

We begin to see everyone as our sister and brother and we begin to love everyone unconditionally. We begin to accept everyone the way they are and we asks no changes of anyone. We begin to experience a wonderful feeling of oneness with every person and living thing. The concept of feeling separate from other people disappears and with it, any feelings of loneliness.

On this higher level of consciousness, often called the inner self, the higher mind or self-realization, we feel calm and content and we experience an almost constant happiness and joy. Herbert Benson, M.D., defined this state as the relaxation response, the opposite of the fight or flight response. When both mind and body are relaxed, immunocompetence is maximized. Risk of catching a cold or flu is minimal and the severity and duration of any infection that might occur is reduced to the minimum. Risk of getting cancer and most other diseases is also at the lowest possible level.

Furthermore, studies have shown that within an hour of switching from fear-based to love-based beliefs and thoughts, the ability of the immune system to manufacture antibodies is dramatically increased. For example, a 1983 study by Dr. David McClelland, a Harvard psychologist, tested the immune reactions of one hundred volunteers after they were first shown a movie about Mother Teresa depicting love, humor and compassion, and then another about Hitler depicting hate and violence. Results clearly showed that positive emotions created by watching Mother Teresa boosted the presence of antibodies in the volunteers' saliva while negative emotions resulting from the Hitler movie suppressed antibodies.

The Faith Factor

At this point, you may be wondering whether you must lead an exemplary life, be good and go to church to stay free of colds and flu. And anyway, aren't you getting into a lot more than you may have bargained for? Is it worth the trouble of screening out negative beliefs and thoughts just to get over a cold more quickly? Wouldn't it be easier to put up with the cold and soothe the symptoms by popping a few cold-remedy pills available at the corner drugstore?

The answer, of course, is that while adopting Positivism might seem a rather large order merely to get over a single cold, its long term benefits are far more expansive.

If you've been averaging three or four prolonged colds each winter, Positivism can reduce your exposure to cold symptoms to a maximum of three or four days each year. It can dramatically cut the risk of developing a complication such as bronchitis or pneumonia. And it can minimize your susceptibility to cancer and to every variety of viral or bacterial infection.

Positivism is easily learned while relaxing in bed with a cold or flu. It requires no physical effort. Nor does it require that you lead an exemplary life, be good or go to church. Yet it *is* interesting to note that several recent studies have revealed that individuals with strong spiritual faith live longer, healthier lives and experience fewer diseases and infections. For years it was thought that the vegetarian diet of the Seventh-day Adventists was the prime factor in contributing to their freedom from heart disease and cancer. But new evidence is showing that their unflagging spiritual faith and positivism may be an even stronger influence in boosting their health.

The existence of what is being called the faith factor in enhancing immunocompetence is currently being confirmed by a variety of studies. For example, further proof of the power of Positivism in overcoming cancer was recently revealed in a report give by Dr. Lydia Temoshek of the University of California, San Francisco, at a meeting of the American Cancer Society's writers' seminar.

Dr. Temoshek made a twenty-eight-month follow-up study of forty patients with medically-confirmed malignant melanoma, a dangerous skin cancer. When half the patients had died, emotional profiles revealed that those who succumbed had twice the levels of anger, hostility, depression, dejection, tension-anxiety, fatigue, inertia and confusion as those who survived.

Dr. Temoshek concluded that upbeat emotions determine a cancer patient's chances for recovery. Commenting on the Temoshek studies, Dr. Wallace Clark, Jr., of the University of Pennsylvania reportedly said that it offered the strongest evidence in favor of Positivism yet.

Mind Over Immunity

Put together, all of these studies, and discoveries within the field of psychoneuroimmunology are clearly and definitely showing that we can consciously choose to have a strong and competent immune system and be relatively free of viral infection (and cancer) by believing and thinking positively, by staying calm and relaxed in body and mind, and by visualizing ourselves as already being the healthy, positive, competent person we want to be.

At any time, we can consciously choose to switch from seeing the world through the fear-based belief system of the lower mind and we can perceive it instead through the love-based belief system of the higher mind.

So the first step is to restructure our beliefs by replacing our old negative beliefs based on past conditioning with new positive beliefs that are more appropriate to the present moment in our lives. For example, past events may have programmed us to believe that the only way to have security is to build a fortress of money. While it may still be prudent to provide for a possible rainy day and for financial security in our old age, it is much more appropriate to recognize that life offers an unlimited abundance of love and goodness and that we need no longer continue to look at everything from a position of lack.

At this point, you may also be asking how you control your awareness. For a start, close your eyes and place your awareness on the big toe of your right foot. Now shift your awareness to your left elbow. Wasn't difficult, was it?

Now imagine a large electric wall switch in the middle of your brain. The down position is marked FEAR, the up position LOVE. Whenever you recognize yourself perceiving the outside world through a filter of fear-based beliefs, visualize the switch in the down position. Hear a loud clang as you move the switch to the up position. Then raise your awareness to the higher mind and view the world through a filter of love-based beliefs.

The fact that Positivism has been endorsed by highly-accredited doctors from top-ranking university medical schools testifies that this is the most powerful tool ever devised to strengthen the immune system. By simply placing our awareness on a higher consciousness level, we are simultaneously giving ourselves a pep rally and determining to have a happy, hopeful, optimistic and confident outlook.

What are these love-based beliefs with which we can restructure our belief system so that we start seeing the world in a positive way? First discovered by yoga philosophers in the forests of India 4,000 years ago, these precepts of universal wisdom have been added to by Greek, Roman and Arab thinkers and by modern pioneers such as Ken Keyes Jr., and Vernon Howard.

Positivism can be instantly achieved by mentally adopting and practicing the following precepts of esoteric wisdom. Perceiving the world through a filter of these beliefs liberates us completely from depression, fear, worry, loss, envy, anger, guilt, stress and all the other fear-based emotions that cause us to upset ourselves and be unhappy.

THE PRECEPTS OF POSITIVISM

1. Inner peace is the goal of life. Do and acquire only things which will maintain and deepen our inner peace. Cease desiring superficial excitement and stimulation. Lasting happiness comes only from contentment. When we are content and at ease, both body and mind are calm and relaxed.

2. Forgiveness is our primary function in life. So forgive everyone, now and forever, whom you feel may have caused you harm at any time. From now on, forgive instantly, on the spot, anyone whom you believe may be threatening you in any way, or pushing your buttons.

3. The way to achieve peace and forgiveness is to stop judging and condemning others. Judging and condemning is nothing more than a surface habit which is easily broken when we forgive everyone and love everyone unconditionally.

4. Live only in the here and now, in the present moment. As we let go of the past, we release all guilt and resentment. And fear disappears as we let go of our concerns about imaginary problems in the future.

5. Realize that the *real you* is not your ego but your higher mind and that its essence is love. Therefore, you *are* love. The ego is totally concerned with animal instincts linked with your body and arising from fear of lack and based on getting and receiving.

6. Realize that giving and receiving are the same. When you give and help others, you will receive back an abundance of love and other good qualities.

7. Love everyone unconditionally (including yourself) and accept everyone as they are without requiring others to

change. (Naturally, children have to be led and guided.) But always remember that you cannot become upset or angry when your awareness is on a higher consciousness level. By allowing only positive thoughts and beliefs, we cannot be upset by anything that others may do or say. If there's something we don't like about another person, the answer is to change our own beliefs so that we perceive the other person without upsetting ourselves.

8. Experience a common oneness with every living thing and regard everyone as your brother or sister. See the higher mind in others rather than their lower ego-mind.

9. Act without seeking a reward—seek not the fruits of your actions. Don't expect to be rewarded for everything you do. Be willing to help others without expecting anything in return, not even a "Thank you."

10. Cease seeking fame, wealth, prestige, recognition, praise and other strokes to swell the ego. Be willing to live unknown and to make your wants few.

11. Experience constant abundance. See no scarcity or lack. Be a millionaire of love and goodness and share your abundance with others. When we focus our awareness on the here and now, we find we always have everything we need to enjoy the present moment. As a result, we can stop wanting and experience immediate contentment.

12. Break attachments to possessions. We don't have to give everything away. But recognize that circumstances can change and we may not always continue to own the things that currently belong to us. Consider, instead, that we are given the use of these things for a while and that we should be willing to share this use with others. If, eventually, we no longer possess them, we can let them go without any feeling to loss. (This does not mean we should give or loan money to financially irresponsible people.)

13. See every problem as leading to a wonderful new opportunity. As one door closes, another door opens. Re-

call that every adversity contains the seed of a greater opportunity. So surrender all problems to a higher power for an answer while you continue to live without worrying. Feel as though a higher power is guiding your life, living your life for you, and even thinking your thoughts for you while you enjoy living without stress or dis-ease.

14. Problems are solved by staying calm and by listening to an inner voice or intuition or gut feeling for guidance. Be careful not to let negative feelings guide you. We must not allow negative feelings to run our lives and determine our choices. We can always tell when we are being run by the lower ego-mind because to receive genuine guidance, we must be perfectly calm and relaxed with our awareness on a higher consciousness level and free of any negative emotions. So try to avoid acting and making choices unless you are completely calm and relaxed.

15. Always be open and truthful. Do not repress or stifle any negative emotions but avoid pouring out your negative feelings on others. Bearing this caveat in mind, do not conceal your inner feelings.

16. Focus only on the best in everything and everybody and overlook their lesser qualities.

17. Never compare yourself with others or with their acquisitions or achievements. And don't look back and compare yourself with how you used to be. Keep your awareness in the present.

18. We can only win when everyone else wins also. Compete only with your own excellence but not with other people.

19. Be flexible and flow along easily with life. Avoid rigidity and holding strong opinions. Accept whatever you cannot change and adapt to it.

20. Accept complete responsibility for whatever you say or do and cease to blame others for whatever happens to you.

21. Avoid using these words: "I, me, my and mine; should

and ought; perhaps, may, might and try; good or bad; and right or wrong."

22. Realize there is no such thing as absolute security. The closest thing to security is to maintain high-level wellness through sound nutrition, exercise and Positivism, and to learn a job skill that is in demand.

23. Being alone or by yourself, or being single, is not the same thing as feeling lonely. We feel lonely when we begin to think that no one needs us. Yet millions of married couples feel so miserable they would prefer to be single. And millions of Americans who must share their homes with others would prefer to have the privacy of being alone. So feel thankful that you have the privacy, and the freedom from spats, that others long for.

24. Whenever you are upset by something that seems to have gone wrong, tell yourself, "It doesn't matter!" The only meaning anything has for us is the meaning we choose to give it. When we are upsetting ourselves over the meaning something has for us, we can restore inner peace by changing that meaning. For example, a woman was extremely upset because her son had decided not to go on to medical school but to join a spiritual commune instead. When she told herself, "It doesn't matter," she let go of the expectation that her son would become a doctor and she accepted that it was all right for him to become whatever he chose to become.

25. Don't expect the world to treat you with fairness and justice. Either exists only in the mind of the beholder.

26. See yourself as a medium for the spread of love and service. Feel that your life is being guided by a higher power (intuition). By staying calm and relaxed, you will always be guided towards doing the best thing and making the best choice—the "best" being that which is most beneficial to you and all others involved. Thus your wel-

fare will always be provided for and there is absolutely nothing to worry about.

Upbeat Emotions Ensure
Swift Recovery From Colds

By restructuring our old inappropriate beliefs with these positive new beliefs, it is virtually impossible to entertain a negative thought. And if a negative thought does appear on our inner movie screen, we can easily learn to recognize it and slide it off.

Without a negative thought we cannot experience a negative feeling. And without a negative feeling we cannot become depressed, fearful, unhappy, angry, anxious, resentful, guilty or frustrated nor can we experience any kind of downer or negative attitude or mood.

"Change your thoughts and change your life," is the slogan of the Science of Mind movement. As long as we are calm and relaxed we can change our thoughts in a second. But once a negative emotion is triggered, it can take hours or even days before we can calm down and become rational once more.

The emotional component in every case of cold or flu is now clear. Invariably, it consists of the same chain of events. By perceiving the world through negative beliefs, a negative thought arises which sets off a negative feeling which triggers the fight or flight response. Stress mechanisms are then put into effect that suppress the immune system and cause us to feel lonely, depressed, helpless, tense, uncomfortable and upset.

Yet each of us has the personal power to block this health-destroying chain reaction by refusing to think a negative thought. By doing so, we may not only prevent or lessen the symptoms of a viral infection. We may also prevent cancer, an ulcer, hypertension, rheumatoid arthritis or any one of a long, melancholy catalog of stress-related diseases and dysfunctions.

Undoubtedly you will hear such excuses as "I need to get angry so I can appreciate the calm periods" or "We can't feel happy unless we have blue periods to contrast them with." In reality, the only time we need to experience a fear-based emotion is when we are actually threatened by physical danger. Other reasons are mere excuses by people who prefer the stimulation of strong emotions to the seemingly unexciting alternative of inner peace.

If and when you do experience a negative emotion, let go of it as soon as you can. Never repress a negative feeling. The best way to calm down is to take a brisk walk or run or to do push-ups or sit-ups or any other type of vigorous exercise. Immediately you calm down, forgive the person about whom you upset yourself. Then forgive yourself for becoming upset. Take responsibility for what has happened and realize that no other person has the power to go into your mind and upset you. We upset ourselves by reacting when another person pushes our buttons. We can change our buttons by changing our beliefs.

How to Use Positivism to Boost Your Immunity

Many people have read and studied this and similar lore while in bed with a viral infection. Through adopting these precepts of Positivism, and by forgiving everyone and letting go of fear, their immunocompetence has begun to soar.

Since no studies have been made, no one can guarantee how swiftly you will recover from a viral infection by giving yourself an intensive exposure to Positivism. However, statistics show that the healing process is greatly accelerated by a positive attitude. Research has shown that people with a strongly positive attitude recover twenty-five to thirty-three percent faster from *any* kind of ailment, disease or dysfunction, including surgery. And positive people are less likely to become sick in the first place.

To begin bolstering your immunocompetence right now, study each of the twenty-six precepts of Positivism, starting with number 1. Stay with number 1 until you have accepted it completely. Don't go past number 2 until you actually have chosen to forgive everyone whom you believe may have caused you harm at some time.

Before going past number 3, become aware of when your mind chatter is at work judging and condemning others. And don't pass number 4 until you can keep your awareness concentrated on the present moment, at least for a short while. If you get no farther than number 4—which you can easily do in a couple of hours while resting in bed with a cold—you will have taken a giant step towards permanently bolstering your immunocompetence.

As your thoughts become increasingly positive, in a matter of a few hours white cell and antibody production should begin to soar.

Caution: although Positivism appears to have great potential for preventing cancer and it has been successfully used to bolster medical treatment of all kinds, it has not yet been confirmed as a cure or therapy for healing cancer without accompanying medical treatment. Positivism as described in this book is not intended as a substitute for essential medical treatment.

10 The Relaxation Approach

In Chapter 9 we learned that immunocompetence attains its highest peak when we think positive thoughts that bring us peace of mind.

Researchers investigating biofeedback at the Menninger Clinic discovered that whenever we have peace of mind, the body also becomes completely relaxed.

This led to their defining the law of biofeedback. It states: "Not only does every change in thought cause a corresponding change in body function, but every change in body function is accompanied by a corresponding change in our thoughts and feelings."

By first calming the mind, the body quickly follows suit and it becomes easeful and relaxed. According to the law of biofeedback, this should also work in reverse. And indeed it does. By first relaxing and calming the body, the mind quickly follows suit and it, too, becomes calm and serene. When the mind is calm and serene, our immunocompetence is enhanced to its optimal level.

Researchers quickly realized that we could speed recovery from a cold, flu or other disease by relaxing the body. Several behavioral scientists went a step further and discovered that if, while in a state of deep bodily relaxation, we made mental pictures of our immune system fighting and destroying viruses, recovery was even swifter.

Out of these discoveries was born the psycho-techniques of Deep Relaxation and Creative Imagery. Deep Relaxation is also known as Relaxation Training, Deep Muscle Relaxation or Progressive Relaxation while Creative Imagery may also be called Guided Imagery.

To demonstrate how swiftly and effectively these techniques bolster our immunocompetence, Mary Jasnoski, a Harvard psychologist, performed a test on thirty-two college students all of whom were known to be good at creative imagery. The students were divided into three groups. During a one hour training session, group one, the control group, received no training. Group two practiced deep relaxation and slow-breathing techniques. Group three also practiced deep relaxation with slow-breathing but additionally, they visualized their immune systems as strong, powerful entities that were vigorously attacking weak cold and flu viruses.

Saliva tests were made immediately afterward to measure two immune system components: salivary immunoglubulin cells (which attack upper respiratory tract viral infections) and helper T cells which spur antibody production.

The control group raised neither count. The relaxation-only group boosted their salivary immunoglobulin level. But the group which practiced both relaxation *and* visualization significantly raised the level of both immune system components.

This study, which was presented recently at the Society of Behavioral Medicine in San Francisco, demonstrated that relaxation alone may help fight colds or flu.

But when imagery is used as well, the overall level of immunocompetence is clearly enhanced.

Relaxation and Imagery
Produce Quick Results

These results were accomplished with only a single hour of practice. By staying relaxed, and by practicing creative imagery at regular intervals, these techniques should dramatically shorten the duration of any cold or flu infection. They should also enable the immune system to lessen the severity of symptoms.

These results were confirmed by a similar study at Ohio State University which was reported in *Proceedings of the Society of Behavioral Medicine* (May 23–26, 1984) Researchers divided thirty elderly residents of a retirement home into three groups of ten persons each. The first group received relaxation training three times a week. The second group received personal social contact three times a week. The third group received nothing. Results showed a 32 percent increase in white blood cell count for the first (relaxation-training) group; an 18 percent rise for the second (social contact) group; and a 6 percent drop for the control group. (An increase in white blood cell count signifies increased immunocompetence.)

Deep Relaxation and Creative Imagery are simple do-it-yourself techniques that can be learned in a few minutes while lying in bed. They will boost immunocompetence more successfully than most medical drugs. And they clearly demonstrate that we all do have some control over our bodies and that we need not be helpless victims of stress, disease or prescription drugs.

You will discover that you can relax your entire body at will whenever you choose. You can eliminate all tension and you can guide your Whole Person into the Relaxation

Response. In this calm and peaceful state, your mind thinks only positive thoughts and you are completely liberated from worry, guilt and fear.

The Deep, Slow Breathing Technique

To practice Creative Imagery, we must first enter into a state of Deep Relaxation. So begin by removing your shoes and any tight clothing. Then lie down flat on your back, arms straight and a few inches from your body, while the legs should also be straight with the feet a few inches apart. Support the head with a pillow. You may lie on a bed or on the floor.

Begin by breathing slowly and deeply, in and out, at the rate of six breaths per minute. Fill the lower part of the lungs first before expanding the upper part. Exhale in reverse. Gradually slow the rates of breathing to only four breaths per minute.

Complete at least twelve deep breaths. At this point, your brainwave frequency should have slowed to 8–13 cycles per second, a level of consciousness known as the alpha state.

Deep Relaxation Ends Colds Sooner

You will now be giving yourself silent suggestions. Stay relaxed and realize you are not giving yourself orders. So avoid any intense or compulsive feeling. Just place your awareness on the limb you wish to relax. Silently say the suggested phrases to yourself and create a mental picture of the limb deeply relaxed. You might also try to visualize your limb as made of cotton or strands of wool. In any case, let everything just happen. Don't try to force or hurry the process. If a daydream intrudes, slide the unwanted thought aside and return to your imagery.

Place your awareness on the right shoulder. Slowly repeat the words, "Relax, relax, relax." Keep repeating this phrase as you let your awareness move steadily down your arm to your elbow and on down to the wrist, hand and fingers. As you mentally relax your arm, visualize it deflating as though you were letting air out of an inner tube. Relax your entire arm from shoulder to fingertips. As you repeat the phrase, "Relax, relax, relax," visualize your arm becoming heavy, limp and quiet.

Then, muscle by muscle, go over your entire body. Mentally relax the left arm, right leg, left leg, buttocks, abdomen and neck muscles. After your neck is relaxed, keep your awareness moving up over the scalp to the forehead. Tell yourself, "My forehead feels smooth and unwrinkled. My eyes are quiet. My face is soft and relaxed. My tongue is limp. My jaw is slack." Place your awareness on the respective area as you repeat each phrase several times.

As you make a mental picture of each limb totally relaxed, you are also giving a strong suggestion to the limb to relax. As this technique drains away all leftover tension, you will enter a wonderfully satisfying state of relaxed peace and calm.

Another Deep Relaxation Technique

You can deepen your feeling of relaxation like this. Picture yourself standing at the edge of a deep, transparent spring at least a hundred feet deep and surrounded by a beautiful peaceful garden. Toss a shiny new dime into the water and then watch closely from about three feet away as the dime darts, rolls, flashes and twists its way deeper and deeper into the calm unruffled depths. In about a minute, the dime is resting on the clear, sandy bottom in an undisturbed world of utter peace and tranquillity.

The effects of this mental exercise are almost identical to those you would experience if completely insulated from all external stimuli. To complete your feeling of total relaxation, picture your arms and legs as pieces of old, tired, limp rope. Visualize your body as relaxed as a rag doll. Feel all tightness and tension slip away.

You should now be in a state of total relaxation. Every muscle should feel entirely tension-free. You should be experiencing a peaceful state of consciousness, not thinking of anything in particular.

In fact, you should be experiencing a delicious feeling of detachment from the worries and pressures of everyday living. As you became increasingly relaxed, the mind disassociates from the body and you become unaware that you have a body at all.

How Biofeedback Can Help Shorten Your Cold

At this stage, you can start employing a simple version of thermal biofeedback to become even more deeply relaxed.

Make a mental image of yourself lying on a warm, sunny beach. Visualize plunging your hands into the hot, sun-warmed sand. Place your awareness on your right hand. Feel the heat of the sand flooding into your right hand. Picture your hand as heavy and warm. Simultaneously, repeat the phrases.

"My hand feels heavy and warm. Warmth is flowing into my hand. My hand feels quite warm. My hand is tingling with warmth."

Keep repeating these phrases. You don't have to use the exact words or memorize them. But say essentially the same thing. As you silently repeat each phrase, visualize a clear picture of each suggestion on your inner movie screen. Or just create the visualization out where your awareness is—in your right hand.

In a minute or two, your right hand should begin to tingle and feel warm. When it does, repeat the same thing with the left hand. Once both hands are tingling and warm, you can deepen the feeling by changing your suggestions to include both hands.

"My hands are heavy and warm. Warmth is flowing into my hands," and so on. Visualize both hands as tingling and warm.

You will probably find that one hand becomes warmer appreciably faster than the other. If so, start with this hand. As soon as you feel tingling and warmth in this more suggestible hand, magnify the feeling. then spread that same feeling to the other hand.

You may find you can speed up the warming process by visualizing the red glow of a hot plate or hot coals inside your hands. Or you might visualize your hands plunged into hot water.

Be sure you are in a moderately warm room with a temperature of at least 70°F. Otherwise, keep your hands under a blanket. Never try to force or hurry anything. Just make the pictures and repeat the phrases.

As the blood vessels relax and dilate in your hands, more blood flows in, making your hands heavier and warmer. During this process, you unconsciously sink into a deeper state of relaxation and suggestibility.

At this point, the subconscious is able to accept vivid and powerful images of the state of health (or any other goal) that you wish to give it.

Using Creative Imagery to Battle Virus Infections

If you carried out the handwarming technique just described, you have already used creative imagery successfully. Creative imagery consists of making clear, mental pictures of what you want to happen. You accompany the pictures with silently-worded suggestions. These powerful thought-images then make a clear statement to the subconscious of whatever you wish to achieve. Through regular repetition of these images, you send pictures of your goals deeper and deeper into your subconscious. Gradually, the subconscious releases powerful inner forces that work subliminally to make your goals a reality.

Although we intend to use creative imagery here to speed recovery from a cold or flu, the same techniques can be used to attain any kind of goal, whether it be financial prosperity, or owning a new home or car, or becoming whatever you want to become.

What actually happens is that we circumvent the conscious mind, with all its critical and analytical functions, and we communicate directly with the subconscious. The subconscious uncritically accepts all the thoughts, images, feelings and beliefs we feed into it. All we need do is to give the subconscious a clear, vivid picture of the goal we desire. The subconscious will then motivate the mind-body to make these images real.

In this case, we are asking the subconscious to fortify the immune system and increase its aggressiveness in destroying invading viruses. So for maximum success, it's best to prepare your mental pictures and suggestions in advance. Write down exactly what you want to heal. Make a rough sketch of each mental picture and write out each suggestion.

For example, you will wish to visualize your B cells multiplying into huge armies and then manufacturing billions of antibodies. Imagine a B cell as a white bean. You need only visualize a dozen or so at one time. See each "bean" cell split itself in half and form two new cells. Then see each of these cells divide and become two more "bean" cells. And so on. Then visualize each B cell spewing out small antibodies shaped like darts. Each B cell can manufacture hundreds of antibodies.

Along with this mental image, you can silently suggest: "My B cells are multiplying rapidly." Later, as you picture the B cells manufacturing antibodies, silently repeat: "My B cells are producing billions of antibodies. Each antibody will destroy a cold (or flu) virus."

You can also picture macrophages as large white cells. These, too, you can visualize as dividing and multiplying. Make a similar picture of killer T cells replicating. They are about the same size and shape as B cells.

How to Make Strong, Vivid Images

Always picture your immune system as strong, tough, powerfully aggressive, invincible, indomitable and unconquerable. Make sketches of your killer T cells and macrophages with wolflike fangs and jaws, and of the antibodies with sharp, dart-like points. See them rush at any virus and tear it to shreds.

Or you can symbolize your white cells as fierce white dogs or white tigers or as any fierce and aggressive animal that always wins.

Visualize the cold or flu viruses as small, weak, disorganized and disoriented. Never picture your ailment as strong, powerful, magical, evil, monstrous, gigantic or fear-inspiring. People who have symbolized a cold or flu as a lion or tiger, a giant or a monster, or a powerful spreading tree or rock have proved to be fearful of the ailment and to have a low level of confidence and belief in their immunocompetence.

Next, make a rough sketch of yourself in perfect health, free of all cold and flu symptoms. Sketch yourself as you were at the healthiest, fittest time of your life. Draw yourself loping along a beach, inhaling great quantities of pure air through unblocked nostrils. Feel complete faith in your ability to destroy any invading virus or bacteria.

Create clear, strong, vivid pictures of your white cells and of yourself in perfect health. Not only see yourself running along a beach but feel, hear, smell, taste and touch the scene. Experience each sensation. Smell the salty tang of drying seaweed, hear the scream of gulls and the roar of surf, feel the sea breeze in your face, the sun on your body, and the grains of sand under your bare feet.

How to Give Strong, Powerful Suggestions

For maximum success, suggestions should always be positive and phrased in the affirmitive. Use the pronouns *I* or *we*. Phrase each suggestion in the present tense as though your goal were already accomplished. Instead of saying, "I will overcome this cold, say, I am free of all cold symptoms." Instead of, "My white cells and antibodies will destroy all invading viruses," say, "The cold or flu has already disappeared and I feel terrific." Use positive action verbs like *I can, I am, I feel* and *I believe*. Never use words like *try* or *attempt* or *perhaps* or *possibly*. All messages to the subconscious must be absolute.

Since feelings intensify images, tell yourself how it feels to be free of a stuffed-up nose, or to have a throat no longer sore, or to be free of a hacking cough. Tell yourself, "I feel wonderful, great, happy and pleased. It feels terrific to be free of that sniffling nose and sore throat. Robust health is now mine to enjoy." Describe the end result you want and, as far as possible, phrase all suggestions as though the desired result had already been achieved.

If you prefer, you can think your suggestions instead of silently phrasing them. This may heighten results.

Otherwise, keep suggestions short and simple. During

creative imagery, repeat each suggestion at least four times. As you say each phrase, picture it and experience it.

Few people are unable to create mental pictures. If you appear to have difficulty, however, write out your suggestions several times each. While writing, you will probably see the image you desire clearly portrayed on your inner movie screen.

The Seven-Step Creative Imagery Process

Now that you have the mental pictures and suggestions ready, you can begin creative imagery. Start by practicing the deep relaxation techniques described earlier until you have attained the deepest possible state of relaxation. Allot fifteen minutes to a creative imagery session and divide it into the following stages.

1. Visualize the cold or flu you want to get rid of. Make it appear weak and disoriented. Visualize thousands of spherical-shaped viruses trying to enter the cells in your nasal passages. (30 seconds).

2. Visualize any medical or herbal supplement, food, exercise or other natural therapy that you are using and watch it boosting the numbers and aggressiveness of your white blood cells. Alternatively, visualize the medication or treatment soothing an afflicted area and reducing inflammation and discomfort. (75 seconds).

3. Visualize your immune system massing in your nose and throat for an all-out attack on the viruses located there. For about a minute, visualize your macrophages and T and B cells replicating in huge numbers. Then see the B cells manufacturing antibodies. Spend thirty seconds visualizing white cells and antibodies from all over your

upper body moving to your nose and throat and massing there for a huge attack.

Then imagine squadrons of B cells firing wave after wave of antibodies at the already reeling viruses. See the viruses flying apart as each antibody strikes home. Next, see hordes of rough, tough killer T cells charge the remaining viral invaders, chewing up and destroying all that remain. Finally, see the huge macrophages sail in and mop up the debris, chewing up the remains of millions of viruses. (8 minutes).

4. Visualize your nose, throat and other afflicted areas as already healed and restored to health. (90 seconds).

5. Visualize yourself in perfect health. (75 seconds).

6. Picture your life's goals as fulfilled and visualize a good self-image. (75 seconds).

7. Congratulate yourself for having taken part in your own recovery. Tell yourself you are feeling terrific. The cold or flu is already gone. Maintain a strong positive feeling. (75 seconds).

If your visualization is finished before the allotted time is up, start over and visualize it again. Repeat the visualization as many times as necessary to fill the allotted time.

End the session by repeating the classic Coué suggestion: "Every day in every way I feel better and better." As you say the words, feel yourself well, cheerful, optimistic and filled with new energy.

11 The Prevention Approach

Through a few simple precautions, we can reduce risk of catching a cold or flu by approximately 80 per cent.

Most colds are caught by hand contact: by first touching the hand or face of a person who has a cold or flu and then touching your own face, nose, mouth or eyes.

To minimize risk of catching a viral infection, avoid shaking hands or kissing anyone who has a cold or flu. Avoid using a phone if an infected person has just used it. The same applies to handling any object that may have just been touched by a cold or flu sufferer.

Above all, keep your fingers away from your face, nose, eyes and mouth. Even if you have just shaken hands with a cold sufferer, unless your hand actually touches your face you are unlikely to catch a cold.

Whenever you have any contact with a cold or flu sufferer, the best precaution is to wash your hands with hot water and soap, then rinse the hands under a running faucet for thirty seconds. This means that a strong flow of water should run over every part of your hands for thirty full seconds. Then wipe your hands with disposable paper tissue. Few viruses should remain on your hands after that.

The precaution is recommended after you have been with anyone who has a cold or flu, even if you didn't actually touch them.

However, cold or flu viruses may also be transmitted through air. Hence it's wisest to avoid contact with sneezers and coughers in crowded places. The most likely locales for catching airborne viruses are where you come into close contact with people, especially in elevators, trains, buses, planes, theaters, restaurants, schools, homes and offices.

Try to limit contact with sneezers and coughers in crowded places. Walk or drive to work if you can rather than go by bus or train. If you find yourself next to a sniffler on an elevator, consider getting off and taking the next elevator. If a friend or relative has a cold or flu, phone them rather than calling in person.

Should you be sneezed or coughed at from close quarters, blow your nose gently but steadily as soon as you can. Take care not to touch your face or nose with your hands. Five minutes later, blow your nose again. Always use throw-away tissues rather than handkerchiefs.

Low Humidity Increases Cold Risk

During winter, use a humidifier or vaporizer to raise the humidity inside your home. Low humidity dries out the mucosa lining nasal passages and increases risk of catching a cold or other upper respiratory tract infection. Being in an air conditioned room in summer also exposes one to low humidity with a similar effect on the nasal membranes.

Sleeping with the mouth open also permits membrane linings to dry out and become more susceptible to viral invasion. Persons with a clogged Eustachian tube, or with sinus problems, are also more susceptible.

A person with the flu should stay home from work. If possible, that person should be restricted to one bathroom and should use only his or her own towel and washcloth. As far as possible, a cold or flu sufferer should be isolated in his or her own room and other family members should stay out. Only disposable tissues should be used. (Kimberly Clark was recently perfecting a tissue called AVERT which contains a chemical which kills all cold viruses.)

It's safest to avoid contact with anyone who has had a cold or flu for a week after the symptoms first appeared. However, a cold becomes contagious approximately twenty-four hours before symptoms appear.

Especially if you live in a small town or community, travel exposes you to new virus strains which can increase your risk of a cold or flu. If you live in a large city, where travelers are frequently importing new virus strains, risk of exposure to a new virus strain through travel is diminished.

Be careful about flying if you have a cold and are susceptible to ear infections. If you have a cold and fly, the plane's descent may aggravate ear pressure. A sharp pain, or a discharge from the ear on landing, may indicate a middle ear infection or even a perforated eardrum. In either case, medical treatment is required.

Otherwise, ear infections can usually be prevented by blowing the nose gently and steadily. Sniffling is another common cause of ear infection, especially in children.

Prophylactic Benefits of Vitamin C

Some researchers claim that vitamin C protects against catching cold. However, the protection lasts for only a few hours. If you are exposed to someone with a cold, or are sneezed at, it has been claimed that you can intercept and squelch a cold by taking 600–700 mg of ascorbic acid as soon as possible. Three hours later, the same dose should be repeated.

The same prophylactic dose could protect you if you anticipate being exposed to a cold virus. Take 600–700 mg of vitamin C just prior to the exposure and a similar dose three hours later.

Don't forget to eat the 80–10–10 way (see Chapter 8) so that your diet contains an abundance of complex carbohydrates (fresh fruits, vegetables, nuts, seeds, whole grains and legumes) and a minimum of fats and oils, meat, whole milk dairy products, eggs, fried foods and refined flour or sugar.

If at least 80 percent of your diet does *not* consist of complex carbohydrates, you should take a good quality multiple vitamin-mineral supplement together with a timed release B-complex supplement containing the entire range of vitamin B components.

To minimize chances of catching cold, most nutritionists advise a daily intake from all sources of: vitamin A 5,000 IU; vitamin C 250 mg three times a day with each major meal; vitamin D 400 IU; vitamin E 100 IU; calcium 750 mg for men, 1,000 mg for women; iron 20 mg; magnesium 400 mg; selenium 100 mcg; (twice a week); and zinc 15-20 mg.

And don't forget to exercise every day.

Avoid Being Alone

Although you can obviously reduce physical risk of catching a cold or flu by staying away from other people, it may not be advisable to do so entirely if it causes you to experience loneliness. Feeling lonely is a type of depression that works swiftly to suppress immunocompetence.

If you commonly experience feelings of loneliness you

may actually reduce risk of catching an upper respiratory tract infection by actively seeking out social contact. This might mean spending more time in the company of friends or family members or attending church or joining clubs or classes where you can meet and mix with other people. Several major studies have documented a clear and unmistakable link between feeling lonely and suppression of the immune system.

Smoking, and drinking alcohol also lower your defenses against viral infections. So does emotional stress, thinking negative thoughts, and feeling depressed or tense and uptight.

Next to avoiding physical contact with a cold sufferer, practicing Positivism and staying relaxed can probably do more to prevent a cold or flu than any other single step. That means staying calm and relaxed, and thinking only positive thoughts. Complete instructions for staying in this desirable state are given in Chapters 9 and 10.

Among things that will *not* give you a cold are exposure to chills or drafts or walking outdoors in rain or cold. Nor, unless you have a fever, will these factors worsen a cold you already have.

However, cold outdoor air could possibly cause nasal membranes to dry out, and it may also reduce interferon production by nasal cells. Nonetheless, the benefits of exercising outdoors in cold weather almost always outweigh such potential drawbacks. And since there are few, if any, viruses in outdoor air, your risk of catching a cold or flu while exercising outdoors in winter is almost zero.

Maintain these simple precautions during the winter cold and flu season and chances are good that you will come through the entire winter unscathed.

Glossary

Alpha state—a calm and relaxed level of consciousness characterized by a slow brain wave of eight to thirteen cycles per second.

Antibody—a tiny Y-shaped protein molecule manufactured by B cells. An antibody is a mirror image of an antigen, the identifying receptor on a cell or virus. An antibody can lock on to the antigen of an invading cell or virus, inactivate it, and identify it for destruction by white blood cells.

Antigen—a surface receptor on a cell or virus. White blood cells recognize antigens on all invading cells or viruses, or in cancer cells, as being non-self or foreign in contrast to those on body cells which are recognized as self.

Antihistamine—a compound used for treating allergic reactions that works by blocking the effects of prostaglandins produced by histamines.

Aspirin—a salicylate which kills pain and reduces inflammation by suppressing an enzyme used in producing prostaglandins.

Asthma—a breathing difficulty caused by constriction of air passages to the lungs.

Autoimmunity—when suppressor T cells are unable to slow down the immune response, antibodies and white blood cells that are supposed to defend the body turn around and attack body cells, usually in joints such as the knees and elbows, frequently causing rheumatoid arthritis. The underlying cause of autoimmunity is believed to be emotional stress.

B cells—white blood cells produced in bone marrow. When an invader enters the body, helper T cells bring a sample of the invader's antigen to B cell populations (which live in lymph glands). The B cells swiftly replicate and begin manufacturing antibodies.

Bronchitis—inflammation of the mucous membranes that line the main air passages of the lungs.

Carbohydrates—all foods of vegetable origin are predominently carbohydrates and supply energy in the form of starch or sugar. See "complex carbohydrate" and "refined carbohydrate."

Cilia—whiplike hairs beating in unison at approximately 600 beats per minute that sweep viruses and other matter trapped in the mucosa down the gullet for destruction by stomach acids.

Clone—an identical copy of a virus or cell with the same genetic instructions. When a cancer cell clones, it produces a tumor composed of identical copies of the original cell.

Complement—a series of protein molecules released when antibodies lock on to the antigens of invading cells or viruses. Complement penetrates the outer coating of the invader, causing its destruction.

Complex carbohydrate—fresh, unprocessed, unrefined fruits, vegetables, tubers, nuts, seeds, legumes and whole grains in the same whole, primary condition in which they exist in nature. They are also known as living foods because all the cells are still alive. They are the only foods that contain fiber.

DNA—deoxyribonucleic acid. The double-stranded helix in the nucleus of all cells which contains the blueprint for reproduction.

80–10–10—a way of eating in which 80 percent of dietary calories are obtained from complex carbohydrates, 10 percent from fat and 10 percent from protein.

Endorphin—an opiate-like polypeptide released in the brain by exercise. It reduces feelings of pain and creates the familiar "high" feeling experienced after exercising.

Enkephalin—a small opiate-like natural polypeptide produced in the brain, similar to an endorphin but with a shorter lifespan.

Enzyme—a protein which serves as a catalyst to speed up specific biochemical reactions within an organism.

Epinephrine—a neurotransmitter (chemical messenger) which increases the body's metabolic rate and constricts the nasal blood vessels.

Eustachian tube—a passage lined by mucous membranes linking the middle ear with the throat.

Fibrinogen—a blood clotting agent released by the immune system to dry up blood and stop bleeding.

Fight-or-flight response—a primitive emergency reaction in which the body prepares itself to fight or run away. It is triggered whenever the mind perceives itself as threatened. Since most negative emotional states are fear-based, they set off some or all fight-or-flight mechanisms. These stress mechanisms continue to simmer for as long as the negative emotion is retained. A major function of the fight or flight response is to suppress the immune system, a condition frequently caused by feeling lonely or depressed. Other fight or flight mechanisms set off by anger and hostility can trigger heart attack or stroke.

Glucorticoid—a steroid hormone secreted by the adrenal cortex which inhibits the immune system during the fight or flight response.

Hayfever—also called allergic rhinitis, is a series of cold-like symptoms resulting from secretion of histamine set off by an allergenic response to pollen or ragweed.

Helper T cells—a white blood cell able to recognize foreign antigens. The cells patrol the bloodstream on a constant surveillance mission and are able to set off and orchestrate the entire immune response.

Histamine—an amine secreted by nasal tissue cells as part of the immune response. Histamine causes inflammation, boosts blood flow in the nasal area, and causes mucosa to secrete copious quantities of mucus.

Holistic—the whole person approach to health and healing which embraces all therapies known to actually work, whether on the physical, mental or spiritual level.

Hydrogenated vegetable oils—polyunsaturated vegetable oils into which hydrogen atoms are injected, radically altering the molecular structure and changing it into a trans-fatty acid, comparable to a saturated fat. Found in many commercially prepared foods, hydrogenated vegetable oils are considered a health hazard by most nutritionists.

Immune system—a complex organization that includes the thymus gland, bone marrow, white blood cells, complement, interferon and antibodies, all dedicated to destroying any invading bacteria, fungi, protozoa, virus or cancer cell. It is the body's resistance, its defense system against infections and cancer.

Immunocompetence—a measure of the effectiveness and competence of the immune system in conquering an invading bacteria, fungi, protozoa, virus or cancer cell. Immunocompetence is enhanced by exercise, sound nutrition and Positivism and is suppressed by counterproductive health habits, junk food and negative thoughts and emotions.

Immunoglobulins—(formerly called gammaglobulins), a class of proteins of which antibodies are composed. Immunoglobulins are found in both the bloodstream and saliva.

Influenza—a severe viral infection of the upper respiratory tract, of which many varieties exist.

Interferon—a lymphokine, or protective protein, released by body cells under attack by invading viruses that serves to immunize neighboring cells against viral takeover. Gamma interferon is released by helper T cells to stimulate the immune response.

Killer T cells—or natural killer cells, are T cells which attack and destroy viruses and all non-self cells, including cancer cells.

Laryngitis—inflammation of the mucous membranes and vocal cords in the larynx or voice box, located in the windpipe, causing hoarseness or loss of voice.

Lymphocyte—a collective name for both T and B cells which arise from the lymph glands.

Lymphokine—chemical messengers released by white blood cells and used for communication between the various immune system components.

Macrophage—large scavenger white blood cells which patrol the blood stream on a constant surveillance mission to kill and eat non-self cells and viruses, and to obtain a sample of their antigens.

Mucosa—mucous membranes that line the interior of all air passages and are rich in mucous glands.

Mucus—a slippery, viscid secretion produced by mucous membranes which moistens and protects the mucosa.

Neurotransmitter—chemical messengers, such as norepinephrine, which provide communication between nerve cells in the brain.

Non-self—not of the body, a foreign invader such as bacteria, fungi, protozoa or virus. Cancer cells are body cells so radically changed that they are no longer recognized as self by the immune system.

Norepinephrine—a type of adrenalin, or neurotransmitter, produced in the brain which increases the body's metabolic rate and stimulates most biological drives.

Phagocytes—large scavenger white blood cells which mop up the debris after an attack by lymphocytes and antibodies.

Pharyngitis—a throat infection caused by either a virus or bacteria. Strep throat, a bacteria-caused disease, is the most common and dangerous form.

Pneumonia—inflammation of the alveoli or air-exchange cells in the lungs. Caused by either a virus or bacteria, pneumonia may arise as a complication of a cold or flu.

Polyunsaturated fat—fats, mostly of vegetable origin, in which the double bonds are still unfilled by hydrogen atoms. Most polyunsaturated fats are liquid at room temperature and occur naturally in nuts, seeds, legumes, grains and avocados; some are found in fish body oils. The largest dietary source of polyunsaturated fats are vegetable oils pressed from grains, legumes and seeds. These oils may oxidize on exposure to air, releasing reactive free radicals capable of causing cancer.

Positivism—a therapy being rapidly adopted in behaviorial medicine, based on thinking and feeling only positive thoughts and emotions. Positivism is the single most influential factor affecting health and well-being and is the most powerful booster of immunocompetence.

Prostaglandin—a powerful hormone-like substance made from polyunsaturated fats and used as a chemical messenger by the immune system to trigger inflammation.

Protein—consists of twenty-two amino acids which, in various combinations, form the building blocks of the body. Animal foods supply whole protein, ready for assimilation by the body but no vegetable food supplies whole protein. Instead, two or more protein-rich vegetable foods, such as beans and rice, must be combined to produce whole protein.

Psycho-Technique—a psychological technique such as sliding a negative thought out of your mind and replacing it with a scene of a beautiful beach.

Pyrogen—a chemical messenger used by the immune system to set off an increase in the body's core temperature to fever levels.

Refined carbohydrate—also called simple carbohydrate, is created when a complex carbohydrate, such as sugar, rice or wheat, is stripped of its germ and cellulose walls and is transformed by refining into white flour, white sugar or white rice. The refining process destroys all fiber and most vitamins and minerals. Only empty calories remain. The missing nutrients cannot be adequately restored by enriching. All types of sweeteners, alcohol and dried fruits are also refined carbohydrates. The body's need for these foods is zero.

Remission—a condition in which the symptoms of a disease abate in force and intensity, either temporarily or permanently.

Rhinovirus—the virus that causes approximately 60 percent of all colds. Over 120 varieties have been identified. Shaped like a soccer ball with twenty different faces, the rhinovirus can shuffle the amino acids in its protein coat so that the surfaces are constantly changing, making it difficult to produce a vaccine.

RNA—ribonucleic acid, a copy of the original DNA genetic instructions from a cell nucleus. When inserted into a cell's polyribosomes, unlimited copies of the original RNA are manufactured.

Saturated fat—fat molecules having a carbon skeleton containing the maximum number of hydrogen atoms. Most saturated fats are of animal origin and are solid at room temperature. They are considered hazardous to health.

Sinusitis—inflammation of the mucous membranes of the sinuses caused by a bacterial or viral infection spread from the nose.

Strep throat—a type of pharyngitis, or throat infection, caused by a bacteria and which may arise as a complication of a cold or flu.

Suppressor T cells—white blood cells which slow down the immune response after it has destroyed invading viruses or non-self cells.

T cells—white blood cells originating in the thymus gland which act as helper T cells, killer T cells, or suppressor T cells.

Tonsillitis—acute inflammation of the tonsils caused by a bacteria which may arise as a complication of a cold or flu. Primarily a child's disease.

Virus—a tiny entity consisting of a package of genetic material enclosed by a protein coat. It is not alive but is able to bind to a receptor in a host cell which then draws the virus inside. Once within, the virus sheds its protein coat and the genetic core replaces the cell's own DNA, allowing the virus to reproduce as many as 1,000 copies of itself before the cell hemorrhages and releases the new viruses.

Bibliography

Alexander, Dale. *The Common Cold and Common Sense.*
Los Angeles: Nash Publishing 1971.

Antimicrobial Agents and Chemotherapy Journal. Zinc
Gluconate for Colds. January 1984.

Bandler, Richard. *Using Your Brain for a Change.* Real
People Press, 1985.

Basu, T. K.; C.J. Schorah. *Vitamin C in Health and
Disease.* Avi Press, 1982.

Bennett, Hal Zina. *Cold Comfort.* New York: Clarkson
N. Potter, Inc., 1979.

Benson, Herbert. *The Mind Body Effect.* New York: Simon & Schuster, 1979.

————. *Beyond the Relaxation Response.* New York: Time
Books, 1984.

Berger, Stuart, M.D. *Dr. Berger's Immune Power Diet.*
New York: Signet Books, 1985.

Bresler, David, M.D. *Free Yourself From Pain.* New York:
Simon & Schuster, 1979.

Burns, David D., M.D. *Feeling Good*. New York: William Morrow, 1980.

Casewit, Curtis. *Quit Smoking*. Para Research, 1983.

———. *The Stop Smoking Book for Teens*. New York: Julian Messner, 1980.

Challem, Jack C. *Vitamin C Updated*. New Canaan, CT.: Keats Publishing, 1983.

Chandra, R.K., M.D. *Nutrition, Immunity and Infection*. Plenum Press, 1982.

Cheraskin, Emanuel; W. Marshall Ringsdorf Jr.; Emily L. Sisley. *The Vitamin C Connection*. New York: Harper & Row, 1983.

Nutrition and the Immune Response. *Dairy Council Digest*. vol. 56, no 2, March–April 1985.

DuChateau, J. Gebal. Beneficial Effects of Oral Zinc. *American Journal of Medicine*, vol 70, May 1981.

Evans, Elida. *A Psychological Study of Cancer*. New York: Dodd, Mead, 1926.

Fabricant, Noah, M.D. *The Dangerous Cold*. New York: MacMillan, 1965.

Ford, Norman D. *Good Health Without Drugs*. St. Martin's Press, 1978.

———. *Natural Ways to Relieve Pain*. Harian Press, 1979.

———. *Arthritis*. Prentice Hall, 1980.

———. *Secrets of Staying Young and Living Longer*. Harian Press, 1981.

———. *Mind-ing Your Body*. Autumn Press, 1982.

———. *Good Night—Sleep Well, Live Well*. Para Research, 1983.

———. *Lifestyle for Longevity*. Para Research 1984.

———. *Formula for Long Life*. Harian Press, 1985.

Freeman, Lucy. *Your Mind Can Stop the Common Cold*. Peter H. Wyden, 1973.

Garrison R.; E. Somer. *The Nutrition Desk Reference*. New Canaan, CT.: Keats Publishing Inc., 1985.

Glassman, Judith. *The Cancer Survivors; and How They Did It*. New York: Doubleday, 1983.

Groverland, Jack. *Miracles Made Easy*. Miracle Publishing 1985.

Hammer, Signe. The Mind as Healer. *Science Digest*, 1984.

Hoffer, Abram, Ph D., M.D. *Orthomolecular Nutrition*. New Canaan, CT.: Keats Publishing, 1978.

Howard, Vernon. *Pathways to Perfect Living*. Stein & Day, 1975.

Imperato, Pascal James, M.D. *What to do About the Flu*. New York: E.P. Dutton & Co., 1976.

Jaffe, Dennis T. *Healing from Within*. New York: Knopf, 1980.

Jampolsky, Gerald M.D. *Love Is Letting Go of Fear*. Celestial Arts Press, 1979.

————. *Teach Only Love*. New York; Bantam Books, 1983.
————. *Goodbye to Guilt*. New York: Bantam Books, 1985.

Jarrett, Peter. The Wars Within. *National Geographic*, June 1986; vol 109, no 6, 702 + .

Keyes, Ken. *Handbook to Higher Consciousness*. DeVorss & Co., 1979.

Knight, Allan, M.D. *Asthma and Hayfever*. New York: Arco, 1981.

Lesser, Michael M.D. *Nutrition and Vitamin Therapy*. New York: Grove Press, 1980.

Locke, Steven and Mady Hornig-Rohan. *Mind and Immunity*. New York: Institute for the Advancement of Health, 1983.

Lynch, James T., Ph. D. *The Broken Heart; the Medical Consequences of Loneliness*. New York: Basic Books, 1977.

Mervyn, Leonard. *Vitamin C: Enemy of the Common Cold*. Thorsons Publishers, 1983.

National Academy of Sciences. Diet, Nutrition and Cancer. *National Academy Press*, 1982.

Pauling, Linus, Ph.D. *Vitamin C, the Common Cold and the Flu*, revised edition. New York: Berkley Publishing, 1983.

Public Citizen Health Research Group Health Letter. *Colds, Part I, Stuffy Nose, Fever*. November–December, 1985. 4–5. *Colds, Part II, Cough, Sore Throat*. January–February, 1986.

Régnier, Edmé, M.D. *There Is a Cure For the Common Cold*. Parker Publishing 1981.

Science News. A Cure for the Common Cold. Vol 127, May 11, 1985, 292.

Science News. Viral Closeup; in from the Cold. Vol 128, September 21, 1985.

Siegel, Bernie S., M.D. *Love, Medicine and Miracles*. New York: Harper & Row, 1986.

Simonton, O. Carl; Stephanie Matthews-Simonton; James Creighton. *Getting Well Again*. Los Angeles: Jeremy P. Tarcher, 1978.

Stone, Irwin. *The Healing Factor: Vitamin C Against Disease*. New York: Putnam, 1972.

Thomas, Lewis. *The Youngest Science*. New York: Viking, 1986.

U.S. News & World Report. Viruses: New Look at an Old Enemy. May 12, 1986.

Weiner, Michael A., Ph.D. *Maximum Immunity*. Boston: Houghton, Mifflin, 1986.

About the Author

Norman D. Ford is a medical researcher and self-help author and an expert in holistic therapies. He has written for *Prevention* and *Bestways* and other well-known health magazines and has lectured extensively to health groups and organizations. He has authored more than forty books in the fields of retirement, leisure and health. Norman Ford practices what he preaches and his lifestyle is built around the Whole Person health practices described in this book. Norman Ford lives in the Texas Hill Country and is an avid hiker, bicyclist, swimmer and vegetarian. He is an accredited member of the American Medical Writers Association.